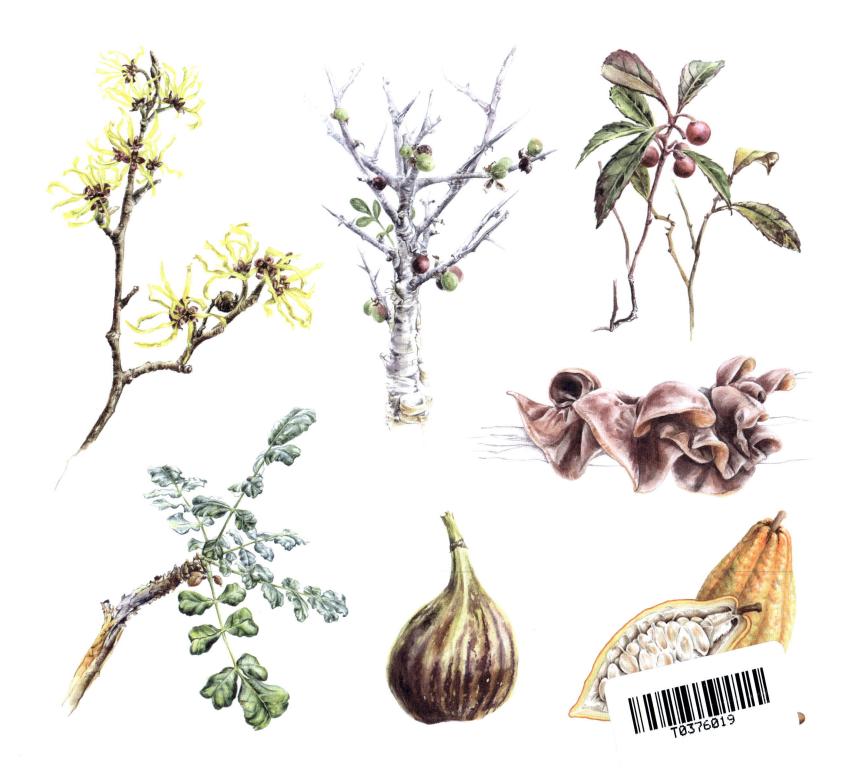

HERBOLOGY
A Physic Garden Pharmacy

CATHERINE CONWAY-PAYNE

with illustrations by Jacqui Pestell MBE
and photography by Kate Soltan

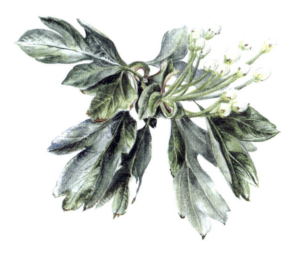

For James Fraser Mansell

(1969–2020)

*You are a thousand winds that blow,
you are the diamond glints on snow.*

ISBN: 978-1-910877-50-0

© Royal Botanic Garden Edinburgh, 2023
Published by the Royal Botanic Garden Edinburgh
20A Inverleith Row, Edinburgh, EH3 5LR
rbge.org.uk

Proceeds from sales of this book will be used to support the work of the
Royal Botanic Garden Edinburgh.

The Royal Botanic Garden Edinburgh is a Non Departmental Public Body (NDPB)
sponsored and supported through Grant-in-Aid by the
Scottish Government's Environment and Forestry Directorate (ENFOR).

The Royal Botanic Garden Edinburgh is a Charity registered in Scotland (number SC007983).

EDITED BY
Frankie Mathieson, Royal Botanic Garden Edinburgh

DESIGNED BY
Caroline Muir, Royal Botanic Garden Edinburgh

PRINTED BY
McAllister Litho Glasgow Limited

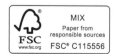

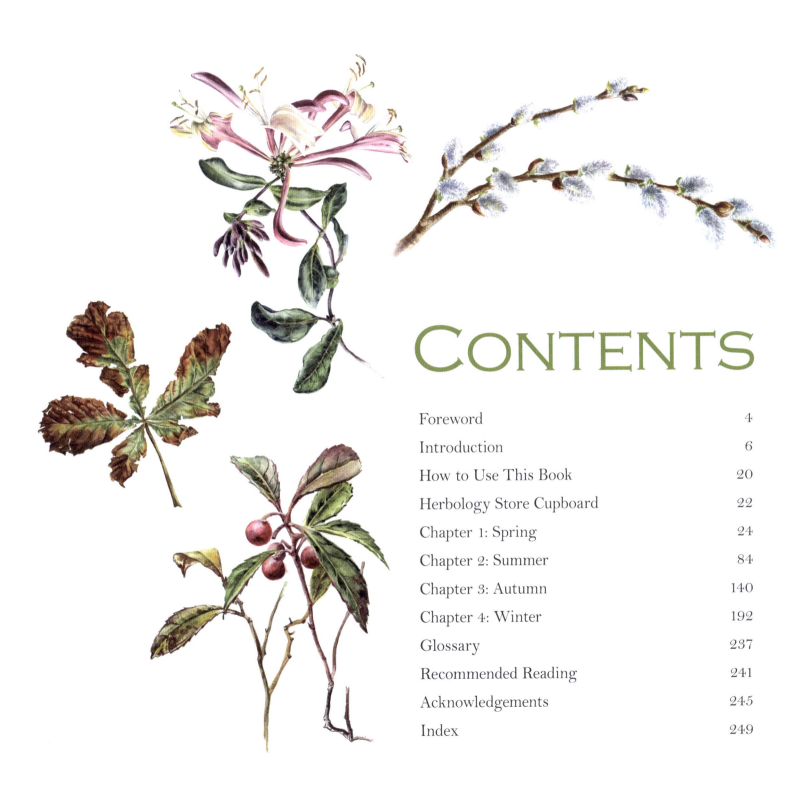

CONTENTS

FOREWORD

Over the centuries, few endeavours have woven together the strands of science, art and history as harmoniously as the study of herbology. Humans have long turned to plants and fungi for sustenance, health and well-being, and in this exquisitely illustrated book we embark on a botanical journey that not only celebrates the rich history of herbal knowledge but also pays homage to the enduring mission of the Royal Botanic Garden Edinburgh – to explore, conserve and explain the world of plants for a better future.

The origins of the Royal Botanic Garden Edinburgh can be traced back to the establishment of a physic garden in 1670 by physicians Sir Robert Sibbald and Andrew Balfour, within the grounds of Holyrood Palace. Since then, it has blossomed into a beacon of botanical research, discovery and education, fostering a deep connection between humankind and the botanical world, enriching our understanding of plant diversity and its myriad roles in shaping and sustaining our lives. The Garden's 17th-century objectives of building a collection of plants for research,

health and education continue to be at the heart of its work today and are beautifully reflected in the pages of this book.

The journey into herbology is one that transcends time, spanning ancient civilisations, medieval apothecaries and modern laboratories. This book artfully presents herbal knowledge intricately linked to the seasons, interweaving the threads of cultural traditions, scientific inquiry and horticulture. The enchanting illustrations and vivid photographs serve as a poignant reminder that herbology is not merely a scientific pursuit but also an artistic expression that invites us to explore and marvel at the value and intricacy of the natural world.

In the 21st century, plants retain immense relevance in the realms of medicine and healing. They serve as invaluable sources of remedies and inspiration for pharmaceutical advancements. Centuries of traditional medicine practices and modern scientific research have unveiled a wealth of plant-derived compounds with potent therapeutic properties, forming the foundations of countless medicines used to treat various ailments and enhance overall well-being. Moreover, plants not only provide us with medicinal drugs but also offer valuable insights into the development of innovative therapies. By harnessing the power of plants, we can unlock new pathways to healing and make remarkable strides in medical advancements.

However, it is disheartening to note that around 40% of plant species on our planet face the looming threat of extinction. This biodiversity crisis necessitates immediate action to safeguard humankind's future welfare. The intricate relationship between plants and humanity extends far beyond their medicinal value, as they provide essential resources such as food, clean air and ecosystem stability. Preserving plant biodiversity is crucial for sustaining ecosystems, ensuring food security and mitigating climate change. Recognising the urgency of this crisis, we must take decisive action to protect and restore endangered plant species, conserve their habitats and promote sustainable practices that foster harmony with nature. This commitment is fundamental for a sustainable future, enabling us to maintain a harmonious balance with the natural world and safeguard the well-being of present and future generations.

Catherine Conway-Payne's contribution to the Royal Botanic Garden Edinburgh and its work extends far beyond her authorship of this book. For nearly two decades, she has inspired and engaged students, staff and visitors with her profound knowledge and passion for herbology.

I invite you to immerse yourself in the pages of this enchanting book, allowing the rich tapestry of herbology, the green pharmacy and the enduring legacy of the Royal Botanic Garden Edinburgh to captivate your senses. May it ignite within you a deep appreciation for the botanical wonders that surround us and inspire a renewed commitment to cherish and protect our natural environment, which continues to nurture and sustain us.

Simon Milne MBE FRSE FRGS
Regius Keeper

INTRODUCTION

This book hopes to capture, and celebrate, a moment in time at the Royal Botanic Garden Edinburgh ('the Garden') through the sharing of a selection of herbal remedies currently being made by our herbology groups within the Garden itself. These recipes (or 'receipts' as they were formerly known) are taken from among our favourite pieces of 'green pharmacy' that we practice.

Green pharmacy describes any form of botanical medicine or herbal remedy making. It lies at the very heart of the study and practice of herbology and physic garden horticulture, where you literally grow the ingredients (the *Materia medica*, 'materials of medicine') of your chosen recipes from seed.

An expression of nature's potentially vast and perpetually burgeoning medicine chest, green pharmacy affords an abundance of therapeutic and quite often (although not always!) delicious preparations, many of which will have their origins in, and be steeped in, traditional herbal medicine making from around the world.

The Diploma in Herbology handbook, composed for those hoping to embark upon this rather unique programme of studies at the Royal Botanic Garden Edinburgh, begins with: 'There has never been a more auspicious time to study all things "green", to learn how to work as one with nature, understand the precious therapeutic potentials of medicinal plants and how to nurture the earth that sustains them.'

These words, written over a decade ago at the point at which this book goes to print, are a thousand times more poignant in this present moment of our history than they were back then, because it is now not simply 'auspicious' to study all things green and to learn how to work as one with nature – it has become prescient upon us all.

The very nature of herbology (literally the study of herbs) is so expansive that once you are immersed within this facet of botanical learning, you cannot help but become aware of its inherently curative and dynamic spirit. It enables every individual to appreciate, embrace and respond as effectively as they can, and in however small and seemingly inconsequential a way, to so many of the catastrophes that currently threaten the natural world and this precious, breathtakingly beautiful planet that we all share and inhabit.

This is herbology's moment, and for the generations who hopefully follow, it may perhaps come to be viewed as a period of great holistic change and life-sustaining initiative. Herbology is experiencing a renaissance of thinking and practices, and of 'reconnections with nature' – from global conservation and sustainability to the more local nurture of healing (physic) gardens and home pharmacy.

Our herbology programme is embedded in the Royal Botanic Garden Edinburgh's rich medicinal history and the content of this book is in many ways a simple reflection of this.

An homage in no small part to the Garden's 17th-century origin as a physic garden, this book references and draws on extracts from four other highly complementary publications that date from around this same period, all intimately linked in the nature of their content to the Garden's own past and present study of medicinal botany. These written works are: *Hortus Medicus Edinburgensis* (1683) by James Sutherland, *Complete Herbal* (1653) by Nicholas Culpeper, *Kalendarium Hortense* (1664) by John Evelyn and translated extracts from the first edition of the *Edinburgh Pharmacopoeia* (1699).

THE *EDINBURGH PHARMACOPOEIA* OF 1699

That the Royal Botanic Garden Edinburgh was founded as a physic garden in 1670 is widely known; what is less well known is that a now relatively obscure little leather-bound book, long housed within the library archives of the Royal College of Physicians Edinburgh (RCPE), holds the secrets to many of the formulations that these botanicals were later destined to make. This is the very first edition of the *Edinburgh Pharmacopoeia*, in whose compilation Sir Robert Sibbald, one of the original Edinburgh Physic Garden founders, was undoubtedly involved. The *Pharmacopoeia* was effectively a 'medicine maker's handbook' to accompany the catalogue of medicinal plants in *Hortus Medicus Edinburgnesis* that was drawn up by James Sutherland, who curated the original garden.

Thanks to Sutherland we know which medicinal plants were being grown in Edinburgh during the latter part of the 17th century, which may be regarded as something of a golden age of herbalism. Similarly, thanks to the work of Sibbald and his unfaltering determination to bring the *Pharmacopoeia* into print, we know how many of these same physic garden botanicals were being used to make medicines.

Both of these intimately connected medicinal plant publications are the first of their kind in Scotland and afford a unique historical insight into the then still closely aligned worlds of plants and medicine. Originally published in Latin, the contents of the *Pharmacopoeia* have remained relatively inaccessible to most for over 300 years. However – with the kind assistance of the RCPE and the dedicated work of one research associate from the Garden, Robert Mill – the work in its entirety has now been translated into English; several extracts of which are being shared, for the first time, within the pages of this book.

A Little *Edinburgh Pharmacopoeia* History

Immersed in the tranquillity that ensues from the study of medicinal physic and/or other gardens of a bygone age, it is all too easy to forget that these were troubling times. To study the old 17th-century maps of Edinburgh and behold what to all intents and purposes appears to be a burgh of delightful green gardens belies nothing of the reality of that particular moment in history. Beyond the sanctuaries of horticulture and the hallowed libraries of academia in Edinburgh there was a great deal of social disquiet and unrest, and it is a somewhat sobering thought to reflect on the fact that the last legal execution for witchcraft took place in Sutherland in 1727.

In the tempestuous years leading up to the appearance of the first rather ornately named *Pharmacopoeia Collegii Regii Medicorum Edimburgensium* (Pharmacopoeia of the Royal College of Physicians of Edinburgh), there was considerable disorder in Edinburgh and the practice of pharmacy fell somewhat drastically into decline and, subsequently, disrepute. There were unsatisfactory shortcomings in the quality, compounding and dispensing of reliable drugs by the Edinburgh apothecaries who were completely unbound by the well-established *Pharmacopoeia Londinensis* (London Pharmacopoeia), whose highly influential content was indeed far-reaching (as may be seen in Culpeper's herbals) but whose actual jurisdiction only extended as far as Berwick, enabling the Edinburgh apothecaries to make as many idiosyncratic and/or dubious variations in their own formularies as they pleased!

It seems there were many protracted discussions among the physicians involved in the *Edinburgh Pharmacopoeia* (1699) compilation over what should and should not be included. It needed to be distinctive but most imperatively up to date, and so over the 18 years it took to come to fruition there were to be many revisions. Some of the more notable remedies that were official in the *London Dispensatory* (1649) were carried over into the *Edinburgh Pharmacopoeia*. One such was the legendary 'treacle water', *Aqua theriacalis* (p. 162).

The actual extent of the *Materia medica* found among the 'simple medicaments' in the first edition of the *Edinburgh Pharmacopoeia* is quite extraordinary and, it has to be said, like no other that would appear subsequently.

Opposite are but a tantalising few with their wonderful Latin names (if given) as they appear in the *Pharmacopoeia*:

- POWDERED TOAD (*Bifo exsiccatus*) – used as a fluid eliminative (don't try at home!)

- OIL OF EARTHWORMS (*Oleum lumbricorum*)

- GARDEN SNAILS (*Limaces cochlea*)

- TINCTURE OF CASTORIUM (*Tinctura castorei*) – beaver scent glands!

- WATER OF FROGSPAWN (*Aqua spermatis ranarum*)

- MOUSE DROPPINGS (*Stercus murium*) – among a selection of other dungs

- DRAGON'S BLOOD (*Gumi sanguis draconis*)

- TOBACCO PIPE CLAY (*Terra cand.*) – literally 'white earth'

- SPIDER'S WEBS (*Telae Aranearii*) – well they had to be there, didn't they?

- VOLATILE SALT OF VIPERS (*Sal volatile viperarum*)

- EAGLE STONES (*Aetites, Lapis aquilae*) – essentially hydrated peroxide of iron, it was believed that eagles furnished their nests with these stones to protect their fledglings, and extraordinary virtues were attributed to them

In the last moments of the 17th century, Sibbald and his fellows of the RCPE had captured a passing era of medicine making that would never come again – in the *Pharmacopoeia* we may find some of the last vestiges of a *Materia medica* that was on the cusp of change. So much of this old and fascinating *Materia medica* was about to fall out of favour and become quite literally written out of the ensuing later editions. It would have eventually faded from the memory and been lost to us with the passage of time but for the safe keeping of the earlier pharmacopoeias themselves, now the sole and precious repositories for the curiosities of bygone medicinal beliefs and practices.

For those remedial substances and compounds with little if anything much to redeem them, their disappearance may not seem such a bad thing – it is, after all, an unfathomable thought that mouse droppings should ever find their way back (intentionally!) into our holistic formulations. That said, some of the other equally unpromising 'simples' (the ingredients of medicine making) of the past have already been destined for rediscovery – the humble snail is one, now enjoying something of a comeback on account of the recently rekindled interest in the therapeutic, generally cosmetic value of their slippery slime.

MATERIA MEDICA OF THE GARDEN, PAST AND PRESENT

FROM *HORTUS* TO HERBOLOGY

It rather goes without say, that one of the greatest perks for the herbology programme at Royal Botanic Garden Edinburgh is the vast array of *Materia medica* (of the purely vegetal kind!) that inherently surrounds it.

This *Materia medica* is comprised of the Garden's many medicinal botanicals that have been coming into its collections since 1670 and are effectively 'on tap' for the studying herbologist. Where else, apart from another similarly placed botanic garden, could you hope to find such a botanical treasure trove? Suffice it to say, Sutherland would have definitely agreed.

We are able to read, in his own words, the significance Sutherland attached to the value of the locally grown medicinal botanicals of the early physic garden in this extract from the introduction to his *Hortus Medicus Edinburgensis* (1683), in which he writes of the 383 medicinal plants in his care:

For now it plainly appears that many of the Simples that were wanting here and there, and yearly brought from abroad, because of their usefulness in Physick, may now by Industry and Culture be had in plenty at home. And it is evident that the Apothecaries Apprentices could never be completely instructed in the Knowledge of Simples (which necessarily they ought to be) before the Establishing of this Garden; for now they may learn more in one Summer, then formerly it was possible for them to do in an Age. And to make the thing easier for Beginners, I have Planted in One corner of the Garden, the Dispensatory Plants in an alphabetical Order.

Sutherland's considerations towards the needs of the apprentice apothecaries and students of medicinal botany – not to mention the care he evidently took to facilitate their learning – says much about his character. It is an endearing thing to discover that his book was apparently on sale in the physic garden at that time – an indication of not only visitor interest in what was taking place there horticulturally but also proof that there were visitors to the Garden even in those earliest moments of its existence – and then we come to realise, on such fundamental levels at least, how very little has changed.

It appears from the extensive *Materia medica* noted in his *Hortus Medicus Edinburgensis* that Sutherland was determined to have on hand as many of the simples as might be in regular usage by the apothecaries as he was reasonably able to grow – and even those he wasn't, such as the gum arabic (noted in his appendix as *Acacia nilotica* (L.) Willd). It seems unlikely that he would have been able to nurture this successfully beyond its natural range without a glasshouse, although it was clearly attempted.

Gum arabic, it would seem, is a fairly desirable piece of *Materia medica*, whatever the period of medicine making. It quickly became an indispensable and much-loved ingredient of one of our most popular green pharmacy preparations, so in many ways we feel a debt of gratitude and quite a deep sense of connection to Sutherland's efforts with this one botanical alone.

THE FORBIDDEN FRUITS OF SUTHERLAND'S *MATERIA MEDICA*

Sutherland's *Hortus Medicus Edinburgensis* reveals many things of intrigue to the eagle-eyed enquiring herbologist on the threshold of determining what their own small herb bed might legitimately comprise. It was with some glee that we discovered on closer reading of *Hortus* that dandelions were being grown as recognised (and most significantly, accepted!) simples within the physic garden of many years ago. Abandoning all the cautionary, contemporary curatorial warnings against this practice to the wind (but hopefully not the wayward downy seed heads), the more hedonistic of our herbologists were keen to do the same and cited this historic precedent as impunity for their wayward horticultural practices. And so, it transpires that dandelions (along with several other forbidden 'weeds') have come to be once more consciously and most carefully cultivated among the living collections of the Garden.

Such wild medicinal botanicals may be found growing in almost carefree abandon within the native heath and woodland corners of the Garden, where the more natural habitats that they enjoy have been faithfully recreated. These precious wilderness sanctuaries afford a valued and rich supply of alternative *Materia medica* for herbology's green pharmacy, beyond that being purposefully cultivated in the dedicated physic garden's herb beds. They have almost become places of pilgrimage for our herbology groups, either on the trail of the first exuberance of remineralising spring greens for 'wild bear's medicine' (any remedy being prepared with *Allium ursinum*), or an atmospheric autumnal fungi foray towards the close of the year.

All our favourite 'escapees' are there, it seems – and as it turns out, nearly all are to be found in *Hortus Medicus Edinburgensis* and the *Edinburgh Pharmacopoeia* too – from the tiniest wood sorrels, primroses, nettles and celandines to the rubberiest of jelly ears – and it all seems like manna from heaven to us!

The collection of medicinal herb beds that now make up what has become fondly referred to as the 'herbology physic garden' (and originally comprised a culinary potager-style herb bed and an appropriately shaded poison herb bed), came under herbology's jurisdiction as soon as it became apparent that our herbology student plots were putting on such a beautiful – if relatively unseen – show and were deserving of a place in the public Garden where they could be more widely appreciated by the many visitors passing through there.

The herbology physic garden remains the sort of working garden of which Sutherland might have approved, as so many of the botanicals being nurtured there are integral to the studies of medicinal botany, organic and biodynamic horticulture and green pharmacy. For our herbologists, being able to grow and gather their own medicinal botanicals within such a setting as the Royal Botanic Garden Edinburgh is a privilege that is only surpassed by learning how to compose their own pharmacopoeia of healing remedies from them.

Nothing, however, quite compares to the unforgettable experience of heading out into the Garden after hours to gather herbs by the light of a waxing full moon – to know that no one else is around, that the gates have been locked for the night and that the Garden is all your own, is really quite something. Only Marley, the Garden's cat, occasionally joins us for these nocturnal botanical perambulations, plus a small legion of ever-curious pipistrelle bats. To be able to explore the magical realm of the Garden at dusk, holding handfuls of intoxicatingly fragrant herbs with a small group of kindred spirits by your side – it doesn't get better than that!

Of course, not all the medicinal botanicals noted as 'officinal species' in *Hortus Medicus Edinburgensis* would necessarily be destined for use in the remedies of the day or be integral components of the *Materia medica* of the *Pharmacopoeia*. For some, such as the witch hazels, the simple 'lateness' of their arrival to the Garden ensured their absence from both Sutherland's collection and the more familiar 'physic' of the day.

Remedies and the *Materia medica* from which they are made, whatever the form, have a great propensity to fall in and out of favour – their appeal and popularity being in many ways attributable to, and an often-bemusing reflection of, the prevailing attitudes and times from which they have emerged and are most closely associated with.

Even from among the relatively small selection of remedies chosen for this book, it has been fascinating to learn which have endured, which seem to have only been around for a comparatively short period of time but have an ancient provenance, and which have been all but lost altogether – whether they faded gradually over time, or were snuffed out almost overnight with the dawn of a more 'enlightened thinking' and the therapeutically defining parameters of what has become known as the 'pharmaceutical age.'

Many of our best-loved remedies – such as the simplest extracts, unguents and honied confections, have been with us forever, or at least from 'time immemorial', and there is something reassuringly comforting in the simple fact that they have been handed down to us for as many years as they have, with so few (if any) ill effects!

Our most experimental green pharmacy is born from these cornerstones of old and trusted recipes – these are the ones that make up our medicinal heritage, after all. Each remedy that we make carries within it precious lessons to be learnt by the medicine maker themselves. Through the recurring making of these remedies, knowledge is sustained and not forgotten.

BEYOND THE OFFICINAL

It is a revealing sign of the times to see where Sutherland assigned other therapeutic botanicals out with the 'officinal species' list of *Hortus*. Under 'ornamental plants' we have a host of golden daffodils, conspicuous for their abundance in the Garden but not perhaps for their unexpected absence from the early *Pharmacopoeia*. The daffodils especially reveal something of the period's horticultural preoccupations for the latest 'must have' trends and in particular the acquisition of flowering bulbs, which peaked during the 17th century. It also highlights a loss of appreciation for some of the more 'obscure' of the older healing folk traditions that failed to make the *Pharmacopoeia* grade of 1699 – and yet are currently enjoying a tremendous resurgence of interest in contemporary orthodox medicine.

The historic reputation of the daffodil as a purgative, recognised anticarcinogenic and vulnerary that could be applied topically to burns or wounds to induce an analgesic-like numbness was sufficient to encourage the recent pharmaceutical investigations of potentially therapeutic alkaloidal compounds (such as galantamine), found within various *Narcissi*. These have subsequently proven efficacious in the treatment of Alzheimer's, one of the most prevalent and debilitating neurological diseases of our times.

Daffodils are currently being grown in Wales at high altitudes for this very purpose. Apparently, the actions of the alkaloids can be greatly enhanced by the stresses the daffodils experience when grown in the Welsh mountains! Sheep, thankfully, may graze within post-flowering daffodil fields with impunity to their purgative effects. Another earlier spring flower, the snowdrop (*Galanthus nivalis*), has also been found to yield galantamine.

THE *KALENDARIUM*

Around the time of the founding of the Edinburgh Physic Garden (1670), there was a tremendous surge of interest in the study of plants and gardens. The very first botanic gardens had already been founded in Italy over a century earlier, in Pisa, Padua and Florence, to be followed sometime later by the Oxford Botanic Garden in England, which just pipped Edinburgh to the post!

The stage for botanical enquiry had been set and several seminal publications followed – including John Evelyn's *Kalendarium Hortense* (1666), the first gardener's calendar to be published in English and the most widely influential gardener's almanac of its time. Sutherland, therefore, would have been exceedingly familiar with Evelyn's writings, and given that the *Kalendarium* was effectively the 'go-to' gardener's handbook of its day, it would most definitely have been among the books being used and referenced at the Edinburgh Physic Garden.

Evelyn's engaging work, which outlines the yearly tasks to be undertaken by the 17th-century gardener, affords the most remarkable insights into the recommended horticultural practices of the time – albeit some of which would seem better suited to the more temperate, warmer gardens of southern England.

Geographical locations aside, this is a generally precious piece of our horticultural heritage and so much of what is advocated within its pages still holds true. To this end, several extracts from the *Kalendarium* have been faithfully reproduced for your enjoyment throughout the ensuing chapters of this book.

For the contemporary Scots gardener and the herb-bed-cultivating herbologists of our Garden alike, there exists a smaller but highly pertinent alternative calendar, which dates from a little later and may be similarly dipped into, should a 17th-century perspective be required at pivotal points within the growing year: *The Scots Gard'ner* (1683) by John Reid.

Reid was a Scottish gardener who later emigrated to America. As the name of his book suggests, this particular gardener's calendar was quite specifically intended for the gardeners of Scotland and the 'cold, chilled barren Rugged-natur'd ground' that they have to contend with. Here we find no tending of melons or early orangeries but an extolling of the virtues of enclosure, manure, digging and the removal of weeds – all the fundamentals our herbologists need to practise.

While it is Evelyn's *Kalendarium Hortense* that we have chosen to reference here, I highly recommend Reid's book, not least for its appendix of suggested garden fruit recipes that includes pickles, vinegars, preserves of various sorts, liqueurs, and directions for how to make a good 'metheglin' (a honey wine or mead infused with herbs).

We know that Sutherland and Reid were acquainted and the following communication from Reid was sent not long after he arrived in America, confirming his earnest intention to contribute towards the then burgeoning collection of medicinal botanicals that Sutherland was accumulating with enthused gusto in the Edinburgh Physic Garden back home:

> There are a great store of Garden herbs here. I have not had time to inquire into them all, neither to send some of the many pleasant, (tho' to me unknown) plants of this country, to James Sutherland, physick Gardener at Edinburgh, but tell him, I will not forget him, when opportunity offers.

Reid also directs readers of *The Scots Gard'ner* to his learned friend: 'If you would be further satisfied in the varieties of plants, consult the Learned and most Ingenious Mr James Sutherland's Catalogue Phisick Gardener at Edinburgh.'

CULPEPER:
THE COMPLETE HERBAL

Of the hundreds of books that have come into the Garden's herbology 'library' over the years – many of which have been kindly gifted for our use and safe keeping – there are some in particular that have become our most precious and indispensable points of reference. One of these is our oldest edition of Nicholas Culpeper's *Complete Herbal & Dispensatory* (1846), which was generously donated to our collection by our dear friend and herbology follower in Santa Fe, Dr Maureen Mansell.

Carefully turning the hallowed and now rather delicate sepia-tinted pages of this old herbal, it feels for all the world as though you are actually in the company of Culpeper, as in his own

THE

COMPLETE HERBAL,

TO WHICH IS NOW ADDED, UPWARDS OF

ONE HUNDRED ADDITIONAL HERBS,

WITH A DISPLAY OF THEIR

Medicinal and Occult Qualities

PHYSICALLY APPLIED TO

THE CURE OF ALL DISORDERS INCIDENT TO MANKIND:

TO WHICH ARE NOW FIRST ANNEXED, THE

ENGLISH PHYSICIAN ENLARGED,

AND

KEY TO PHYSIC.

WITH

RULES FOR COMPOUNDING MEDICINE ACCORDING TO THE TRUE SYSTEM OF NATURE.

FORMING A COMPLETE

FAMILY DISPENSATORY AND NATURAL SYSTEM OF PHYSIC

BY NICHOLAS CULPEPER, M.D.

words he intimately shares with you all that he knows of the healing botanicals he once sought in hedgerows of the English countryside, along with the many practical remedies that could and may still be made from them.

Within the herbal, each of Culpeper's botanicals is more or less described to us in an introductory profile that includes their distinguishing characteristics, singular virtues, humoral attributes (i.e. whether they were regarded as being hot or cold, moist or dry and to what degree) and the planetary dominion they are generally believed to be most under the influence of. Occasionally though, some of the more common herbs (and indeed the particular steps required to compound them into remedies) are considered to be so familiar and well known to his readers as to require 'no further description' – the audible frustration of an avidly reading herbology student upon reaching such a point in his text can know no bounds!

Culpeper is for many the most memorable of the great Elizabethan herbalists who inhabited the world just a little before the Edinburgh Physic Garden came into being but whose influence would have been one of the most medicinally resounding throughout the 17th century – and is still extraordinarily resonant over 300 years later.

Culpeper acquired a more often than it is not lauded notoriety for his audacious but highly commendable translation of the *London*

Pharmacopoeia from the (then inaccessible to most) Latin into vernacular English.

Published in 1649 as the *London Dispensatory*, with notable additions made by Culpeper himself (he added the all-important and hereto missing uses for each of the medicines), these transcripts became an overnight success among the common populace but incensed physicians who had, up until that point, been the almost exclusive custodians of this highly privileged knowledge.

In this singularly bold act, Culpeper effectively gave medicine back to the people so that the practice of it might be used by and for the benefit of everyone, but especially the poor – unable as they were to afford the extortionate fees of the physicians, or indeed the exorbitant nostrums of the apothecaries who were also to turn against him.

Not to be put off by his detractors, or the accusations of witchcraft that were eventually levelled against him, Culpeper set up his own practice and from there he went on to write *The English Physitian* (1652), which later became known as *Culpeper's Complete Herbal* (1653). Originally sold at only three pence a copy, *Culpeper's Complete Herbal* went on to become one of the most popular books ever published and remains in print to this day.

Culpeper was only 37 when he died, but the remedies and invariably humorous accompanying commentaries found within the pages of his herbals are an enduring legacy of a bygone age of English herbalism of the kind we may never see again; a truly alchemical amalgamation of medicinal botany, astrology and elements of Galenic humoral philosophy.

Culpeper will always be regarded as something of a hero within herbology circles, and it is to him rather than any other historical herbalist that our Garden's own herbologists always seem to return when in need of some traditional, trusted and good-humoured direction for their green pharmacy. For this reason, he is the natural 17th-century herbalist of choice we refer to in connection with some of the simples, remedies and anecdotes chosen for this book.

A NOTE FROM THE AUTHOR: THE GARDEN OF HERBOLOGY

Although I have forgotten exactly when I first walked through the silvered East Gate of the Royal Botanic Garden Edinburgh, I remember perfectly how it felt – like being enfolded in the deepest sense of peace and calm – and as I breathed in the cool and fragrant airs of the beautiful shrubs and trees all around me, I could feel my pace and heart rate slowing. That I had just entered an extraordinarily therapeutic and magical place, I was in no doubt, but I could never have imagined then the destiny that awaited me within the 'inner sanctum' of this particular Garden.

Now, nearly 20 years later, I can honestly say that it has been one of the greatest privileges of my life to be able to walk into work, past railings hung with ornamental currants or round that now-familiar bend in the river, to help create and nurture the Garden's ever-evolving herbology programme.

The following recipes with their associated botanicals are representative of the Royal Botanic Garden Edinburgh herbology contemporary green pharmacy and may be regarded, at least in part, as the Garden's very own home-grown dispensatory.

We hope you enjoy them.

Catherine Conway-Payne
Royal Botanic Garden Edinburgh
Herbology Programme Director

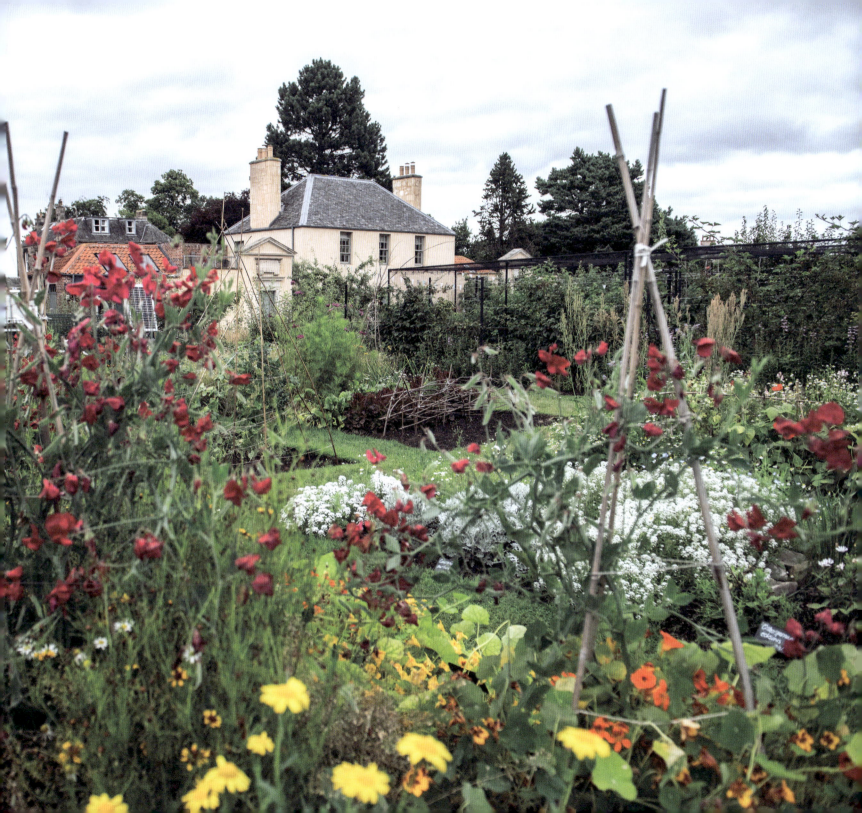

HOW TO USE THIS BOOK

SO, BEFORE WE BEGIN...

Dear reader,

The following herbal formulations are by no means exclusive to the respective seasons into which they have been placed but are organised in such a way because we have found their preparation to be especially rewarding if initiated at this time. Similarly, the choice of the selected botanical ingredients is never better than if gathered from the wild or from carefully tended herb beds at this particular moment in the physic garden calendar.

Also, if we are to start at the beginning, a logical way of presenting herbal remedies might be according to the ever-increasing degrees of complexity required to prepare them – so, here they are, with the simplest of 'simples' coming first! But feel free to pick up this book just as you will, whenever the mood of a season takes you and its full moons are riding high...

WHEN NOT TO USE HERBS

Herbal remedies are generally *not* recommended for the following:

- In the first three months of pregnancy
- For breastfeeding mothers
- For babies under six months old
- When combinations of different drugs are already being taken
- Where there is hepatic or renal impairment
- For those with recognised hypersensitivity and/or a previous allergic reaction to herbs
- For a fortnight prior to surgery

DOSAGES (PLEASE READ!)

Many of the recipes selected for this book are of a tonic, nutritional or confection-based nature. As such, they may be enjoyed a little more freely than those that are distinctively medicinal when specific dosages are recommended.

Please be aware that any dosages given here are for adults only, not for children or the very elderly for whom the concentrations may be too strong or the nature of the remedies themselves (e.g. those that are alcohol-based) not appropriate.

Most of the doses given for the medicinal formulations included in this book are for: one teaspoon (approximately 5ml) to be taken three times daily. Note: 1ml is approximately 20 drops.

While there are standard dosages for most herbal preparations, the potency of any given formulation and its herbs can vary significantly, as can an individual's optimal requirement and indeed tolerance for any given herb and the remedy made from it.

With herbal medicines, less is often more. Many herbalists now advocate the use of only the smallest dropper doses until the body's responses have been gauged.

It is not recommended to use a herb or herbal remedy for an extended period, i.e. more than three months.

DISCLAIMER

The Royal Botanic Garden Edinburgh accepts no responsibility for any allergic reaction or harm that may result from the preparation or use of the remedies shared in this book. For your own and others' safety, please always seek the guidance of a qualified medical herbalist before using any herbs, either orally or topically, as there may be possible contraindications and/or drug interactions.

To find a qualified medical herbalist who may be in practice near you, simply navigate the map and click the blue numbers or red pins here: nimh.org.uk/find-a-herbalist.

Alternatively, you may find the American Herbalists Guild helpful. Here is a link to their register of members: americanherbalistsguild.com/member-profiles.

HERBOLOGY STORE CUPBOARD

We recommend having a stock of versatile equipment and ingredients to hand before attempting any of the recipes in this book. You should be able to find the below items in your kitchen and will find that they crop up again and again in the pages that follow! For ingredients, we have included our favourite suppliers of herbs, soaps, essential oils and other staples.

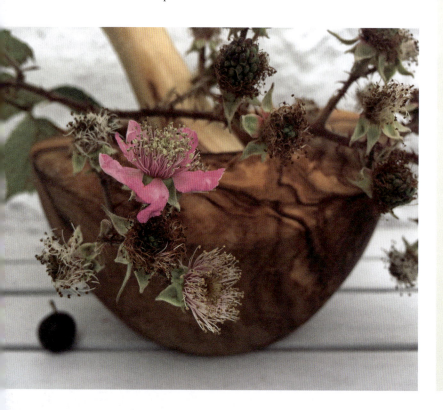

A HANDY LIST OF EQUIPMENT FOR BUDDING HERBOLOGISTS

- BAIN-MARIE – a heatproof bowl or jug that fits inside a heavy bottomed pan
- BLENDER OR GRINDER – a sturdy glass one is ideal
- CHOPPING BOARD
- DEHYDRATOR – stainless steel only. This can be an expensive piece of kit, but could be well worthwhile for drying succulent or juicy soft fruits and berries
- DIGITAL KITCHEN SCALES
- FREEZER ICE MOULDS AND ICE CUBE TRAYS
- JELLY BAGS – for straining (ideally with a stand)
- JUICER – a simple hand-cranked one will do the job!
- LABELS
- MEASURING CUPS AND JUGS – ideally with a 5ml (⅛ oz) minimum, measuring up to 1l (34 fl. oz)
- PESTLE AND MORTAR – stone or earthenware is highly recommended
- SHARP KNIFE SET
- SIEVES AND STRAINERS – a variety of sizes is recommended
- SPATULAS – must be rubber, both narrow and wide bladed
- SPOONS – wooden, metal and measuring spoons (e.g. teaspoon/tablespoon)
- STORAGE JARS/BOTTLES – amber glass, if possible
- TEAPOT OR INFUSER – non-metal is preferred; glass is perfect
- WHISKS – a handheld balloon style and a good electric one

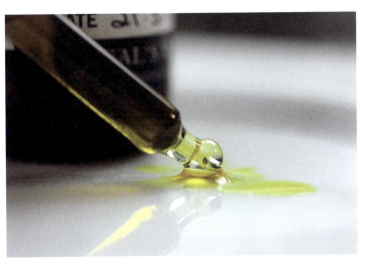

A Trusted Little Green Book of Stockists

- AMPHORA AROMATICS – for aromatherapy and base oils: amphora-aromatics.com.
- AROMANTIC – for a wide range of ethically sourced quality products: aromantic.co.uk.
- G BALDWIN & CO – for quickly dispatched orders of herbs, essential oils and many other botanical products: baldwins.co.uk.
- NAPIERS – for herbal remedies and aromatherapy: napiers.net.
- NEAL'S YARD REMEDIES – for organic, ethically and sustainably sourced herbs and extracts, plus a wide range of natural health and beauty products: nealsyardremedies.com.
- THE SOAP KITCHEN – for butters, bases, oils and pigments needed to make soap: thesoapkitchen.co.uk.

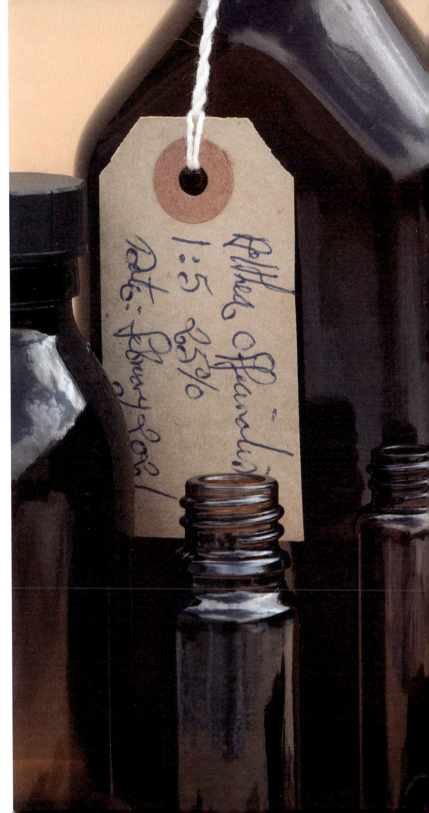

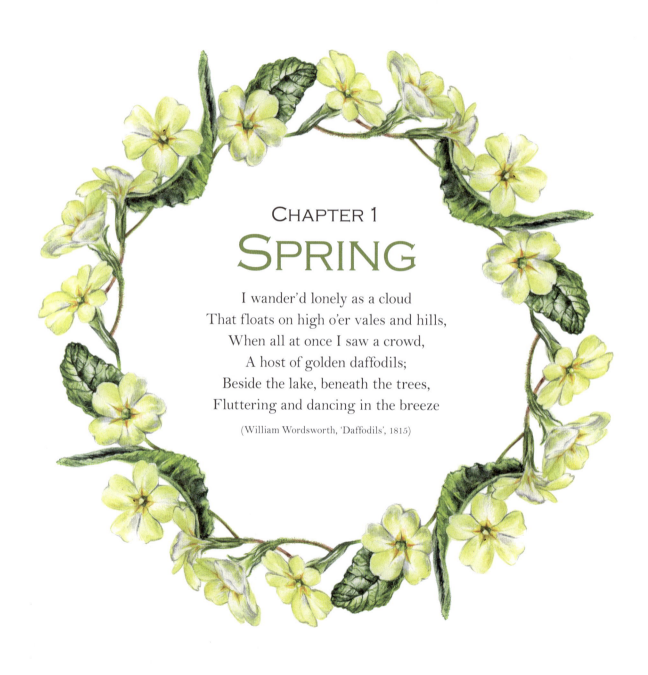

CHAPTER 1
SPRING

I wander'd lonely as a cloud
That floats on high o'er vales and hills,
When all at once I saw a crowd,
A host of golden daffodils;
Beside the lake, beneath the trees,
Fluttering and dancing in the breeze

(William Wordsworth, 'Daffodils', 1815)

The first stirrings within the earth that come with the awakening light of spring are an almost tangible sensation of life's returning energy. This is a time that is full of hope, when the natural world seems to tingle with what the holistic physic gardener will recognise as the 'formative forces' coming into being.

Bulbs buried in trust during autumn or simply at rest in the places they have lain for many years now fulfil their promise, with snowdrops being among the first of the welcome green spikes to emerge from winter ground.

Here at the Royal Botanic Garden Edinburgh ('the Garden'), the refreshing scent of witch hazels fragrance the air – just one deep breath affords such an invigorating rush for the senses.

Within the ancient Celtic calendar, early spring came to be regarded as the 'quickening time' and was celebrated with Imbolc, a fire festival that marked the beginning of the lambing season, fertility and milk flow. The ancient goddess of spring, Eostre, whose sacred creature is often regarded as the hare, was associated with this time and all the natural world waking up after winter.

As the vernal equinox arrives, the warmth of the sun grows and the hours of daylight extend. Birdsong is perhaps never more beautiful than it is now, as the once seemingly hesitant and solitary notes that accompanied the sunrise have become a fully fledged dawn chorus. The equally melodious evensong is a joy to chance upon and hear – endearing affirmations of the anticipated feather-warming times ahead, as nests are made and eggs are laid.

The frogs, similarly caught up in the prescience of the moment, can be heard croaking again and on exceedingly damp nights may be encountered in an almost biblical exodus crossing the Garden and heading purposefully for their favourite ponds.

Catkin-bearing trees such as the common hazel and willows are most noticeable now, with pussy willows resembling soft furry buds. Hedgerows are frothed white with the first of the blackthorn blossoms, interspersed with the golden yellow blooms of gorse – all joyful and ever-reassuring signs that early summer is not so far away – and for pagan hearts, the call of Beltane beckons!

PHYSIC GARDEN DIARY

With extracts from the first gardening book to be published in England, Kalendarium Hortense (1691) *by John Evelyn.*

THINGS TO DO IN THE PHYSIC GARDEN

During the earliest days of spring, there can be considerable periods of time when no work whatsoever can be undertaken in the garden. It is quite simply too cold, stormy or dreich (dull and miserable) to venture forth! But in such wretched times the conscientious gardener might take heart and put to good use those precious moments that brooding clouds on darkening horizons and solid frozen ground present.

Evelyn, in his *Kalendarium Hortense*, suggests:

'In hard weather, cleanse, mend, sharpen and prepare Garden-tools. Now is your season for circumposition by tubs or baskets of earth and for laying your braches [branches] to take root.'

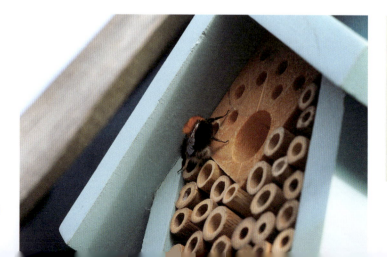

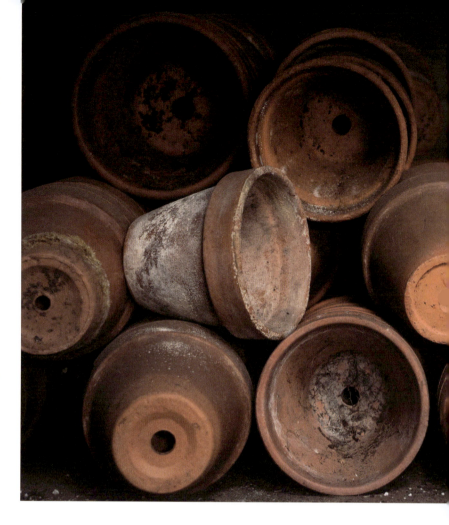

And what better interlude for such good practice could there be? So here begins our own physic garden calendar of things to do:

I.	Clean and repair tools
II.	Clear the cobwebs from sheds, glasshouses and empty planters; organise and tidy them
III.	Dig over the ground
IV.	Earth roots uncovered by any frosts
V.	Preserve botanicals sowed in the autumn from frost and snow

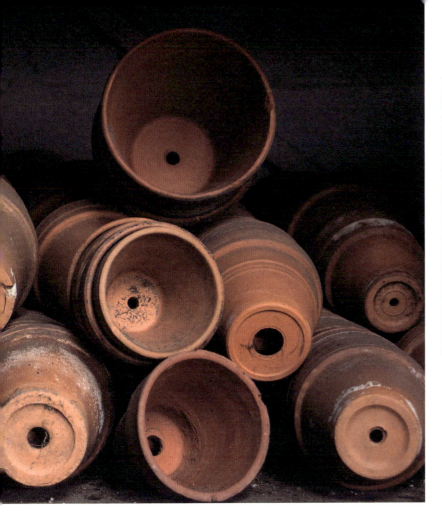

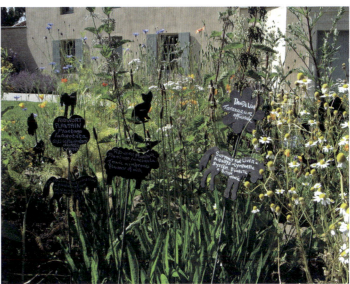

Evelyn expounds on this further to include seeds that are 'in peril from being over-chilled and frozen: covering them and striking off the snow'. In the first of monthly notes for judicious bee husbandry, he writes:

'Turn up your bee hives, and sprinkle them with a little warm and sweet-wort; do it dextrously.'

He also suggests that we should 'enjoy the snowdrops now' – one of the earliest and most precious of possible spring pleasures.

Once the danger of the last snows and frosts has passed, the work in the physic garden truly begins, and the following may take place:

VI.   Prune fruit trees and remove any moss

VII.   Sow early seeds

VIII. Furnish your aviaries with birds 'before they couple'

IX.   Plant hardy kitchen garden and pot herbs. Evelyn recommends: alexanders, basil, beets, black salsify, borage, bugloss, celery, chervil, cress, endive, fennel, leeks, marjoram, parsley, parsnips, skirrets (*Sium sisarum*, a forgotten 17th-century vegetable), sorrel, succory, tobacco and wild celery

X.   Air house botanicals on warm days

XI.   Prune roses. Evelyn notes: 'It were profitable now also to top your rose-trees a little with your knife, near a leaf bud, and to prune off the dead and withered branches, keeping them lower than the custom is, and to a single stem'

XII.   Slip and set lavender, sage, thyme and rosemary

XIII. Turn stored fruit

Evelyn warns against the ravages and 'mischief' of still potentially biting cold easterly and northerly winds. There follows the prudent advice to:

XIV.   Stake up and bind weak plants before they (the winds) 'come to fiercely, and in a moment prostrate a whole year's labour'

XV.   Sow on hot beds 'such plants as are late bearing flowers or fruits in your climate' – enjoy lesser celandines, beds of crocus and early daffodils

XVI.   Sow diverse annuals 'to have flowers all summer'

XVII. Set out and expose plants in pots but 'carefully protect from violent storms of rain, hail and to the too parching darts of sun'

XVIII. 'Mow carpet walks' and trim grass edges

XIX.   Weed herb beds

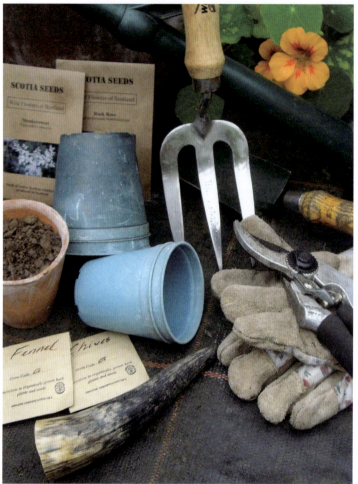

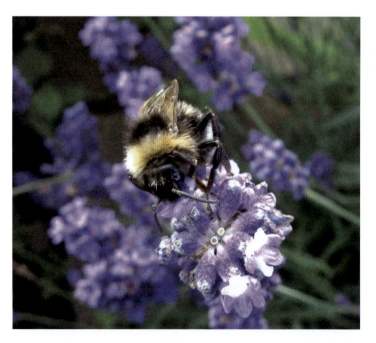

Even for want of a garden, there are many things in Evelyn's diary that may be enjoyed around this time of year. Take a moment to breathe in the gentle fragrances of all the early flowers, buds and blossoms that are appearing almost everywhere they can. Listen to the birdsong whenever you chance upon it, so bursting with gratitude for just the simple gift of life – think on such joys for a moment and allow your own heart to be similarly uplifted in the first truly warm rays of the sun.

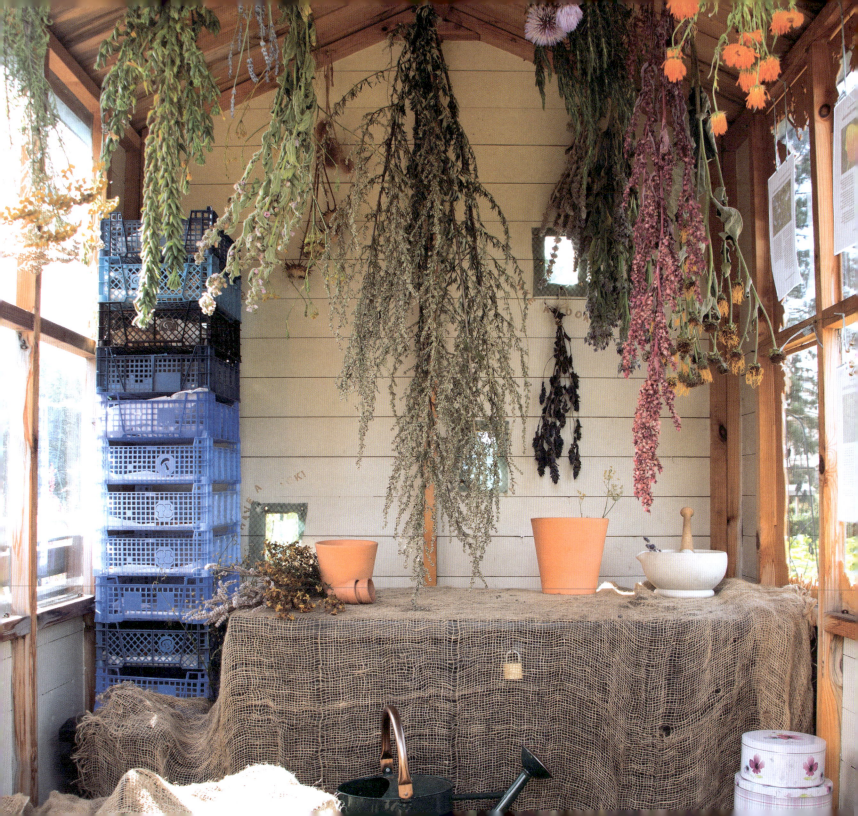

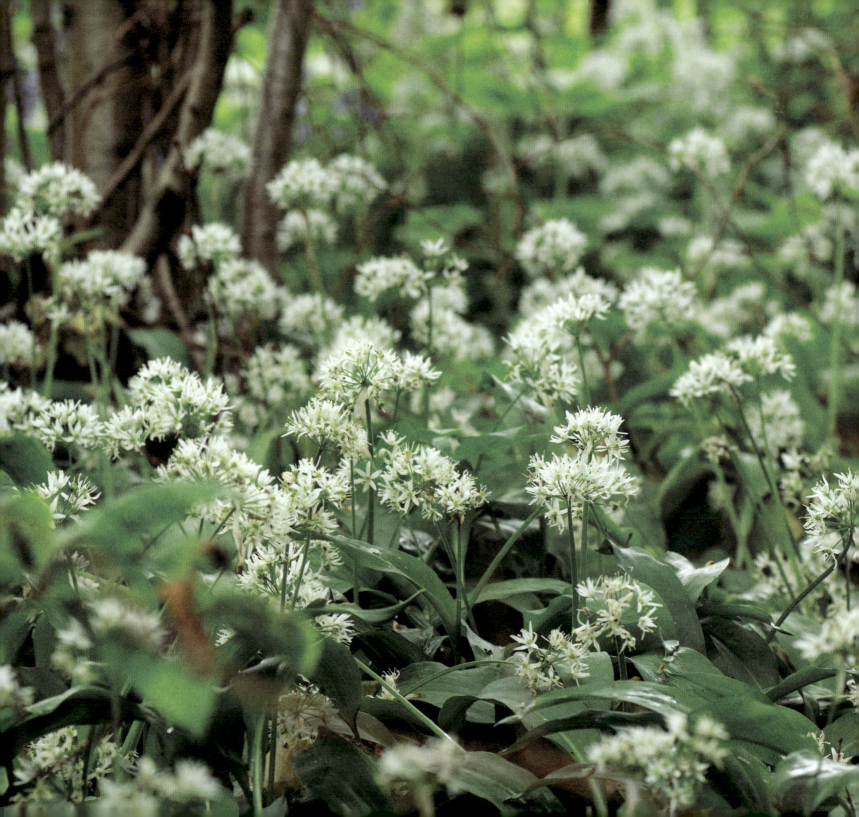

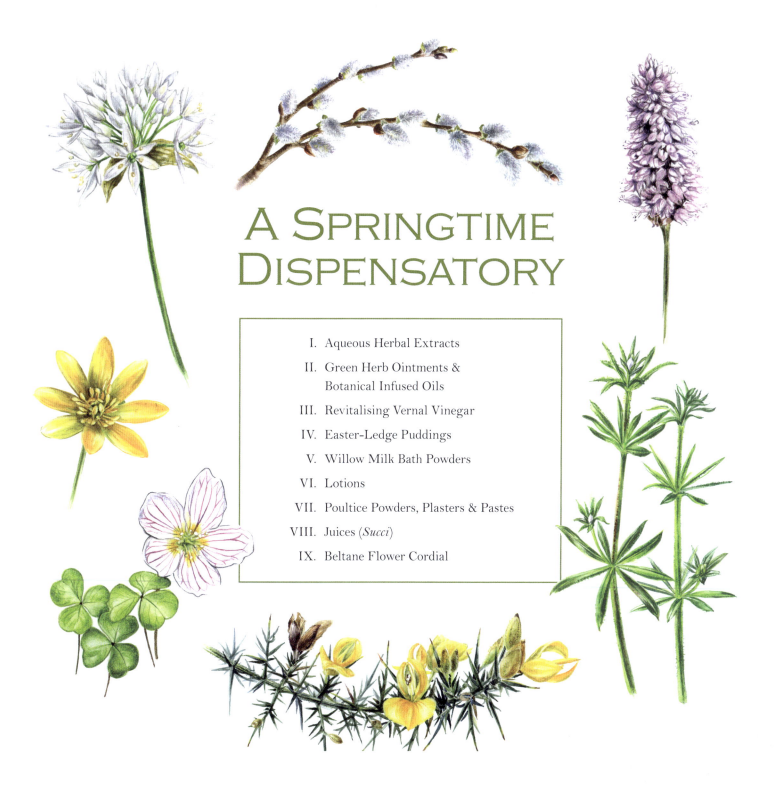

A Springtime Dispensatory

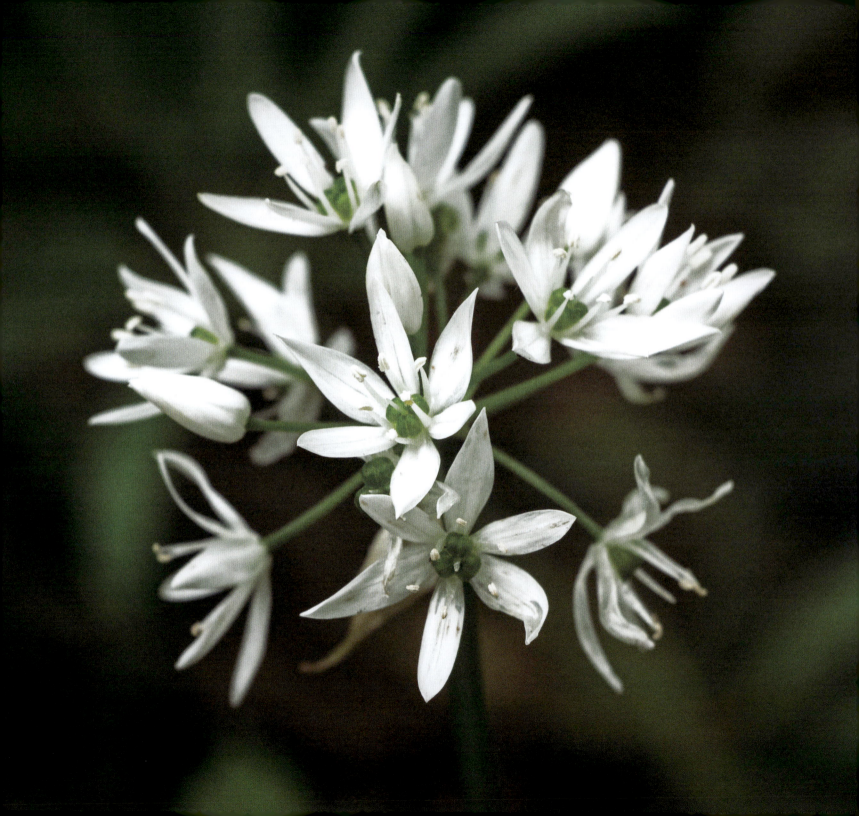

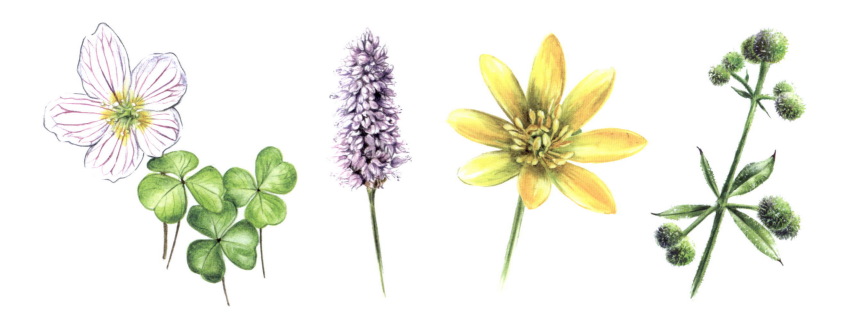

A SAMPLING OF SEASONAL HERBS

Of all the verdant medicinal greens and treasured flowers of early spring, for the Royal Botanic Garden Edinburgh herbologist there are several quintessentially precious (one could argue indispensable) botanicals. Some, such as nettle, dandelion, wild garlic, bistort and cleavers, are among the most eagerly awaited in the 'wild woods' corner of the Garden, from where they are gathered and transformed into our green leaf teas, 'Sticky Willie' waters, revitalising vinegars and herb puddings. Fellow inhabitants of that rather magical faerie realm, like the pignut, wood sorrel, primrose and celandine – often rare and precious finds – remain untouched to be appreciated in other ways, such as through storytelling, rather than being turned into medicines. Others, like the willow, blackthorn and gorse are never more beautiful than when encountered far beyond the Garden's boundaries in their truly untamed and natural habitats.

For herbologists, one botanical is of special significance: the winter blooming witch hazel (*Hamamelis mollis*), one of the very first to return its tangled lemon-yellow knots of fragrant flowers to the Garden. Its beautiful remedies effectively 'book end' the herbology year and so it is included within both our spring and winter chapters.

In this chapter we have also chosen to introduce some of our most valued botanical wound healers, as so many of the remedies made from these require only the simplest of methodologies for their preparation and so this, being the beginning of our book and journey into 'green pharmacy', would seem the most logical place for them.

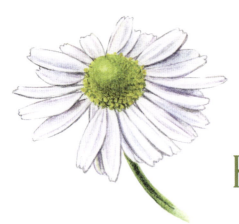

TEN
VULNERARY
HERBS TO TRY

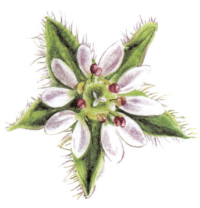

CHAMOMILE
(FLOWER)

German chamomile (*Matricaria chamomilla*) and Roman chamomile (*Chamaemelum nobile*) are excellent anti-inflammatories, which may be in part attributed to the presence of their remarkable water-soluble volatiles. Culpeper (*Complete Herbal*, 1653) references an Egyptian practice (which may or may not have originated in ancient times) of anointing the body with oil taken from chamomile flowers to induce an overnight and therapeutic perspiration. Don't try this at home though, as an immersive application of contemporary (highly concentrated) chamomile essential oil may prove fatal!

CHICKWEED
(HERB)

Chickweed (*Stellaria media*) is, according to Culpeper, under the 'dominion of the Moon'. This quite succulent little herb cools and calms the hottest, most irritated and tickly of tissues. It is a noted antipruritic (anti-itch) remedy – perfect for eczema, psoriasis or sunburn. To make the most of its generally high vitamin C content, a cooling chickweed cream may be prepared from a cold water extract of the herb (p. 40). The juice of the bruised herb or its distilled water (p. 90 – distillates) may also be applied locally or added into cooling lotions.

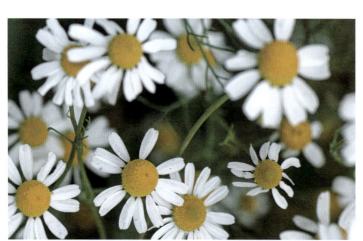

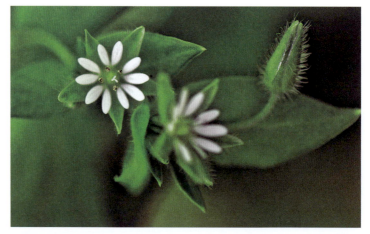

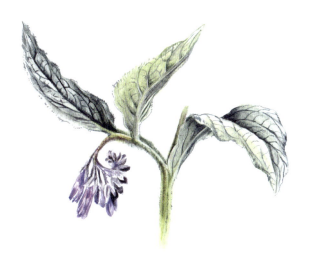

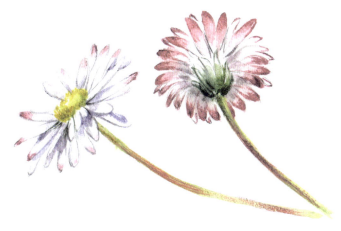

COMFREY
(LEAF OR ROOT)

Comfrey (*Symphytum officinale*) is one of our most mucilaginous botanicals, rich in allantoin and phenolic acids – wound-healing constituents that are easily extracted into herbal formulations and contribute to the herb's justified reputation as an exemplary tissue restorative. Culpeper notes comfrey as a herb of 'very great virtues' and he commends a decoction of the leaf and distilled comfrey water for outward wounds, cuts and sores, with the topical application of the bruised roots being considered especially beneficial for 'ruptures and broken bones'.

DAISY
(FLOWER)

The humble daisy (*Bellis perennis*), formerly known as 'bruisewort' is, as its former name suggests, a remedy primarily suited to bruises. Culpeper notes the use of daisies for 'all bruises and hurts that come of falls and blows', describing a daisy ointment that 'doth wonderfully help all wounds that have inflammations about them'. Thomas Bartram, in his well-thumbed herbologist 'bible' (*Encyclopedia of Herbal Medicine*, 1995) calls the daisy a 'princely remedy for the aches and pains of old gardeners' – one for us all then!

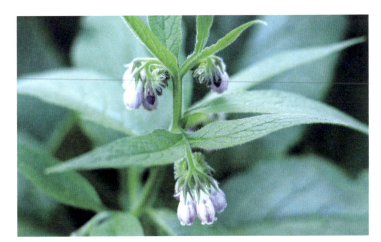

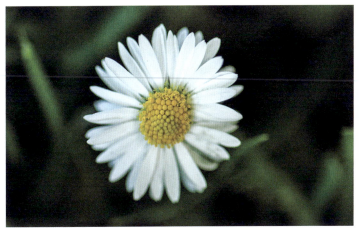

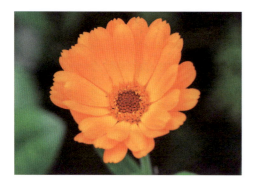

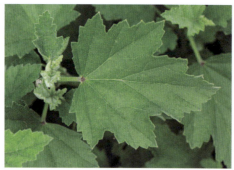

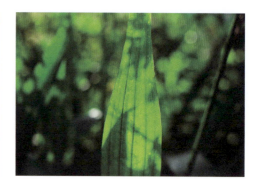

MARIGOLD
(FLOWER)

Marigold (*Calendula officinalis*) is renowned for its ability to encourage the rapid regeneration of damaged cutaneous tissue – *the* quintessential botanical for bleeding wounds, cuts and lacerations – it is an antiseptic, haemostatic and anti-inflammatory remedy. A pharmacy-prepared bottle of 90% calendula extract (for external use only) is a must for any herbal first aid box and may be applied directly to cleansed wounds – much as iodine would have been in the olden days. Culpeper says it is a 'herb of the sun' and that it 'succours the heart infinitely'.

MARSHMALLOW
(LEAF AND ROOT)

Marshmallow (*Althaea officinalis*) leaf and root are both used in herbal healing but it tends to be the root that we utilise to greatest effect within herbology, both as an ingredient of our wound-healing remedies and within our lozenges and cough mixtures (p. 171). Culpeper describes the roots as 'white within' – indeed they resemble bones when peeled and left to dry. Fresh marshmallow root readily exudes the mucilage or 'juice' it holds upon being broken – a silky, soothing and slippery exuberance that imparts the most noteworthy therapeutic effects of the botanical.

PLANTAIN
(FRESH LEAF)

Plantain (*Plantago lanceolata*) is one of our favourite vulnerary herbs. Culpeper recommends plantain as a 'singular good wound herb' – especially when used to heal old wounds and sores. It is the perfect ingredient for a vulnerary green herb ointment (p. 57). Plantain may be nurtured in the physic garden solely for this purpose but also for its seed, which is much loved by birds.

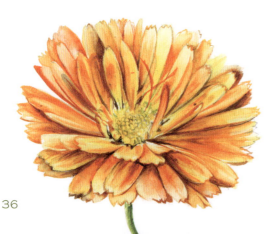

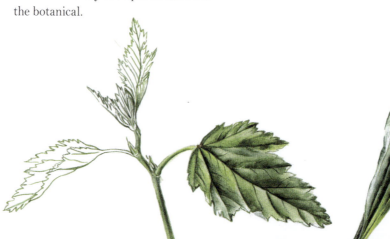

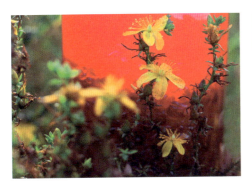

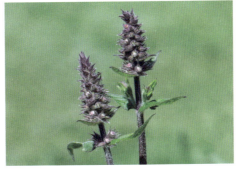

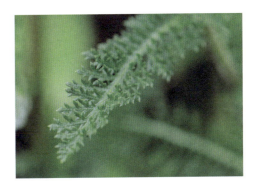

St John's wort
(FLOWER)

St John's wort (*Hypericum perforatum*) is used to reduce inflammation. Formerly known as 'bloodwort', Culpeper describes it as 'a very beautiful shrub…which being bruised do yield a reddish juice like blood'. It is our habit to gather handfuls of the gloriously frivolous flowers to infuse in jars of translucent oil among the hypericum shrubs themselves. The once clear oil gradually becomes a most beautiful ruby red. Highly sought after, the hypericum oil is duly decanted and stored in the fridge for later use in vulnerary formulations such as liniments, creams and our favourite of them all, delicate rose pink tinted balms.

Woundworts
(HERB)

The woundworts (*Stachys palustris* and *S. sylvatica*) are astringent, antiseptic and anti-inflammatory. Perhaps one of the lesser-known or utilised wound herbs of our time, the woundworts often featured in old herbals. Unpleasantly odoriferous, woundworts may be poulticed and applied to wounds. They have a few intriguing little 'secrets' up their leaves too – these include allantoin, betaine (an amino acid that helps the cutaneous tissues stay hydrated, plump and youthful) and choline, a vital nutrient in the formation of phospholipids, which nurture all our cell membranes. No wonder the older herbals loved it – so should we, stinky or not!

Yarrow
(FRESH LEAF)

Yarrow (*Achillea millefolium*) is a noted astringent, haemostatic and anti-inflammatory wound healer. The pulped leaf may be used directly and effectively as a poultice on minor cuts and grazes or infused in a translucent base oil with a little molten beeswax to make the most delightful pale green balm ointment. Culpeper suggests an ointment made of yarrow as a cure 'not only for green wounds, but also for ulcers and fistulas, especially such as abound with moisture'.

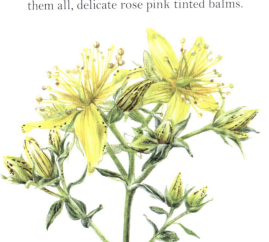

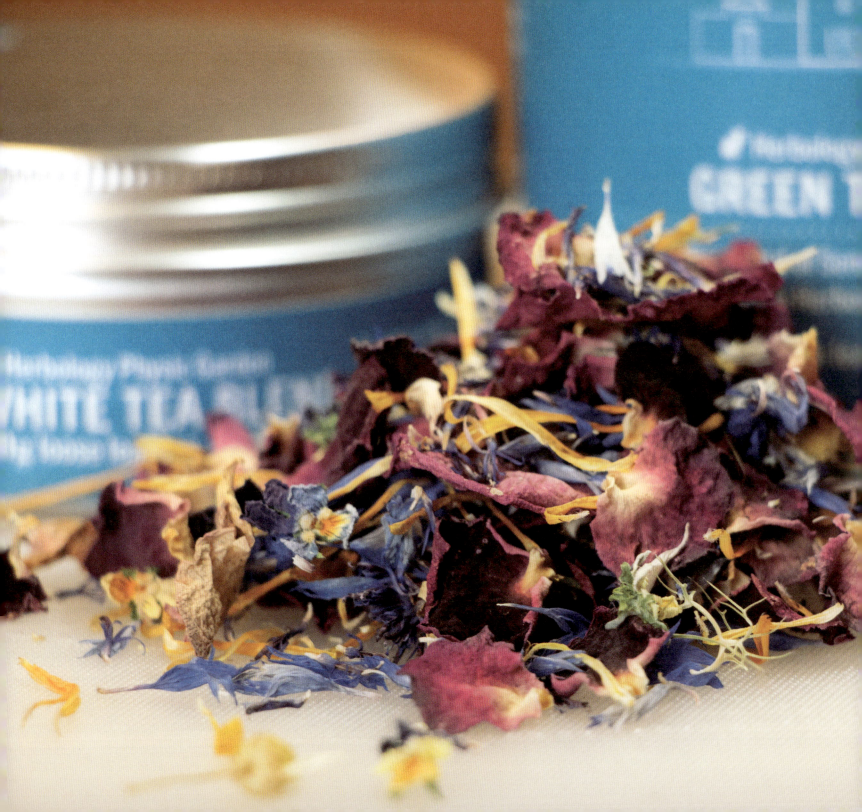

I.

AQUEOUS HERBAL EXTRACTS

WHAT IS AN INFUSION?

An infusion is basically a tea. It is the simplest and purest method of herbal extraction, as it uses only water. Before the highly sought and costly dried leaves of Chinese tea, *Camellia sinensis*, reached our shores, a refreshing cup of tea would be made using mostly locally sourced herbs. Herbal teas (or infusions) may be enjoyed all year round but there is perhaps no better time than spring to gather and prepare the botanical ingredients intended for this purpose – ideally fresh, or dried for later use.

As it doesn't require a lot of effort to prepare a cup of tea, infusions are one of the easiest and therefore most popular of the herbal remedies. Much (if not all) of their appeal depends on how enjoyable they are to drink so it is imperative to choose herbals that can be enjoyed alone or, for the more sophisticated herbal tea maker, cunningly combined to create a truly synergistic blend of memorable botanicals.

Infusions are most appropriate for the following botanical parts:

*   FLOWERS
*   LEAVES
*   SOFT GREEN STEMS

Infusions of barks, roots and seeds are possible, but they generally need to be ground first to break down their harder, woodier and more fibrous structures. It is usually more appropriate to prepare these as decocted extracts.

WHAT IS A DECOCTION?

Decoctions are made whenever the botanical ingredients to be used are hard or woody. This method of preparation ensures that the otherwise difficult-to-reach water-soluble constituents are released into the water. More heat is required for decoctions and the botanicals need to be simmered (or even sometimes gently boiled) in the water. The water-soluble volatiles of aromatic botanicals are all too easily boiled away by this method of preparation so remember to make sure that the pots used for their decoction are always lidded.

Decoctions are most appropriate for:

*   BARK
*   DRIED BERRIES AND FRUITS
*   NUTS
*   ROOTS AND RHIZOMES
*   SEEDS

SOME SWEET ADJUNCTS

Satisfactory sweeteners for infusions and decoctions:

*   HONEY – a must for all those bitter herbs
*   LIQUORICE – dried powdered root (best avoided if you suffer from high blood pressure)
*   RAW CANE SUGAR – use sparingly

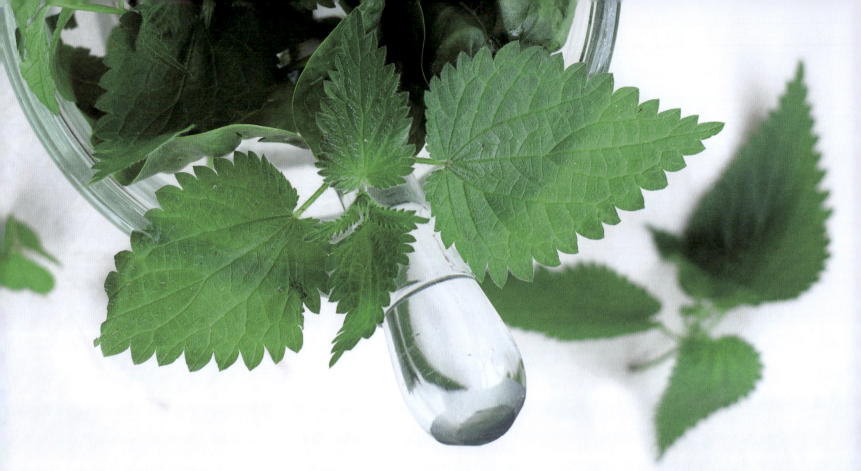

INGREDIENTS & AMOUNTS

Generally, one part of dried herb is equivalent to three parts of fresh – if a recipe recommends one teaspoon of dried herb it can be substituted for three teaspoons of fresh herb. This is because of the higher water content found in the 'green' or fresh botanicals. However, for the purposes of home infusions you can simply double the amount of fresh botanical to dried botanical for a less intense tisane.

To make greater quantities of an aqueous extract (e.g. to fill a vacuum flask with a daily supply), 30g (1oz) of dried botanical or 75g (3oz) of fresh botanical to 500ml (1 pint) of water is recommended (Bartram).

HOT OR COLD WATER EXTRACTION?

Herbal infusions or decoctions may be taken hot, cold or even iced!

If the herbs are very sensitive to heat (either because they are fragile in nature, yield very easily broken-down constituents, or have delicate volatile elements), a cold infusion may be preferred.

For cold infusions the proportion of herb to water remains the same but the infusion should be allowed to stand for several (up to eight) hours in a lidded earthenware pot. Once the liquid is ready, strain out the botanical and use straight away.

STORAGE

An infusion or decoction needs to be refrigerated in a well-stoppered bottle. Water-based extractions do not store well and unless kept completely frozen need to be consumed fairly quickly following their preparation (usually within 24 hours). Whenever possible, prepare only as needed.

HOW TO DRY SPRING GREEN LEAF INGREDIENTS

Medicinally valuable botanicals gathered in the spring, while best enjoyed fresh, may be dried and stored for later use. A wire cooling rack or tray covered in baking parchment is ideal for this purpose. Simply arrange the individual botanical parts so they are not touching and place the whole lot somewhere warm and dry but away from direct sunlight. Turn the botanicals every day, until they are perfectly dry and crunch and crumble when crushed. Once dried, don't be tempted to break the botanicals up into smaller pieces – store them as whole as possible somewhere cool and dry, in airtight dark glass jars or tins and don't forget to label them! Now you have your spring green leaf teas, ready for use at any time. If properly dried and stored, these herbs can easily keep for up to one year.

Author's note: *Please remember that even a simple herbal tea has the potential to exert potent medicinal effects. Do not consume more than three cups of herbal tea a day for any considerable period without the guidance of a qualified medical herbalist.*

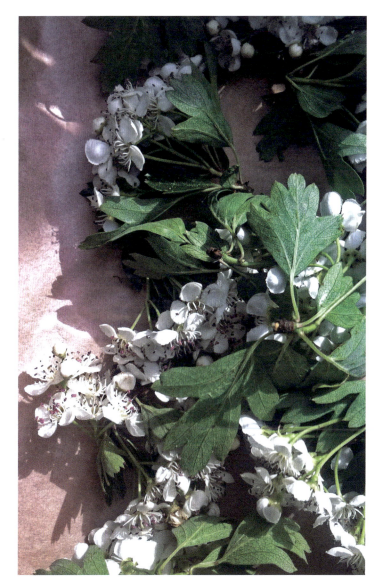

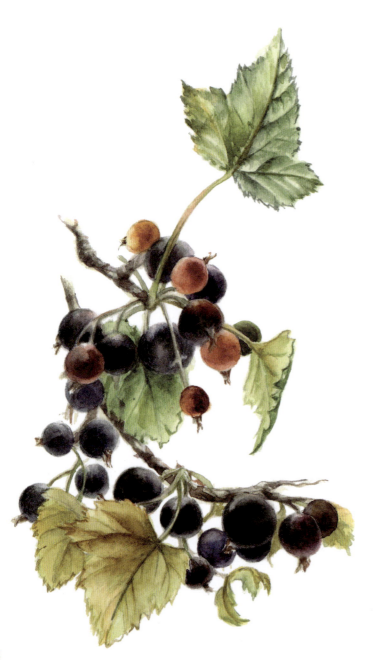

HERBS TO TRY

Here is a small selection of some favourite herbology green leaf botanicals especially for spring, each of which will make a revitalising tea (or decoction) either singularly – referred to as a 'simple' – or combined with others for a re-mineralising, eliminative and detoxifying spring blend. From these few simple 'greens' you will be able to select those that you most like the taste of and those that augment your health.

Author's note: *Gather only the tender parts of each botanical.*

NETTLE (LEAF)
(*Urtica dioica*)

One of nature's finest blood tonics, packed with chlorophyll, iron and vitamin C

PARSLEY (LEAF)
(*Petroselinum crispum*)

Full of immune-boosting antioxidant flavonoids, minerals and vitamins

BLACKCURRANT (LEAF)
(*Ribes nigrum*)

A cooling eliminative, detoxifier and anti-inflammatory – add dried or frozen berries for a delicious antioxidant boost!

Dandelion (leaf)
(*Taraxacum officinale*)

A mineral-rich potent fluid eliminative (don't overdo it with this one!) and detoxifier – add the dried root to make a more bitter hepatic tonic

Cleavers (aerial part)
(*Galium aparine*)

To cleanse, detox and stimulate the lymphatics

Wild 'Bear's' Garlic (leaf)
(*Allium ursinum*)

A natural detoxifier with blood cleansing sulphur compounds, phytonutrients and highly antioxidant phenolics

Birch (leaf)
(*Betula pendula*)

A gentle antioxidant eliminative

Pine (leaf)
(*Pinus sylvestris*)

A potent antioxidant

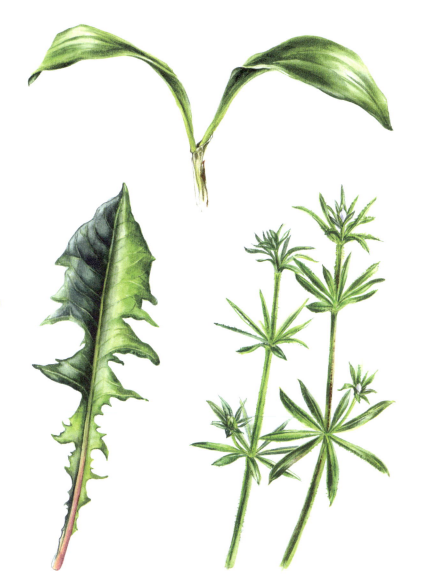

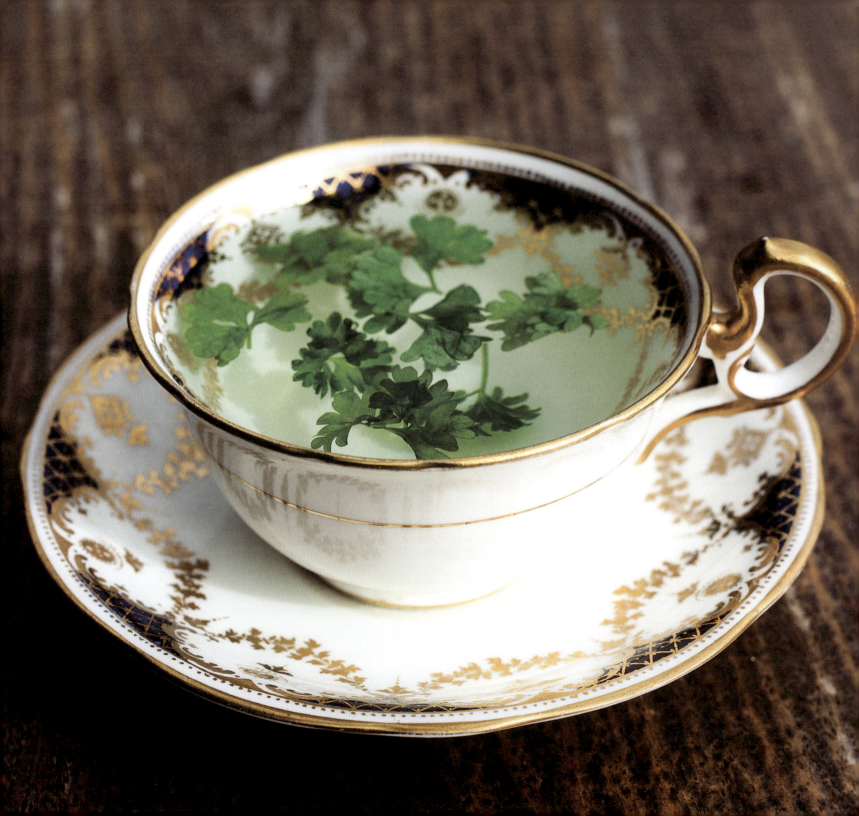

INFUSIONS
RECIPE

INGREDIENTS

1 tsp dried or 2 tsp fresh botanicals (p. 42 – Herbs to Try)

1 cup water or milk for every tsp botanical

HOW TO MAKE

- Warm or chill the pot – china or glass teapots are perfect for herbal infusions
- Add the botanical
- Pour over the water or milk and lid the pot
- Allow to steep/infuse (usually 5–10 minutes)
- Strain and enjoy

HOW TO TAKE

Sip freely – up to three cupfuls a day.

STORAGE

Enjoy immediately or refrigerate and use within 24 hours.

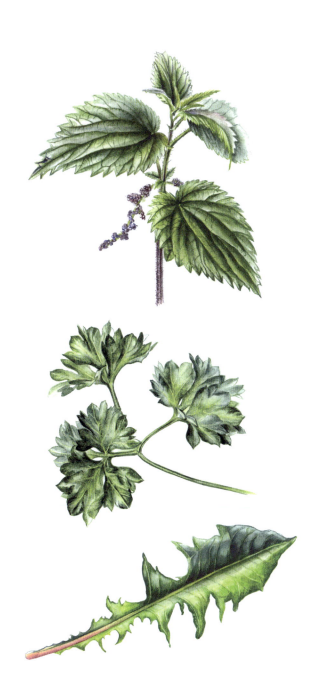

DECOCTIONS
RECIPE

INGREDIENTS

30g (1oz) of preferred crushed or crude botanical
(p. 42 – Herbs to Try)

750ml water

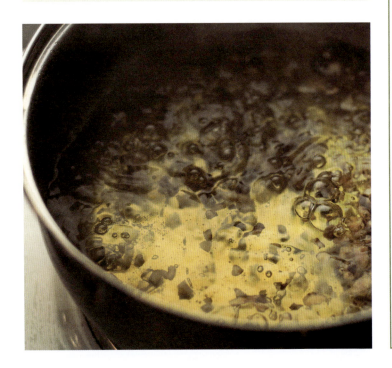

HOW TO MAKE

- Add the botanical to the pan

- Pour over the water

- Bring to the boil and simmer until the volume is reduced by one quarter

- Remember to lid the pan if the botanical holds volatile components

- Strain while still hot and enjoy

HOW TO TAKE

One or half a teacup thrice daily.

STORAGE

Store in a vacuum flask or refrigerate and use within 24 hours.

Author's note: *For really potent decoctions it is best if dried herbal ingredients are first powdered, ground or broken up into small pieces.*

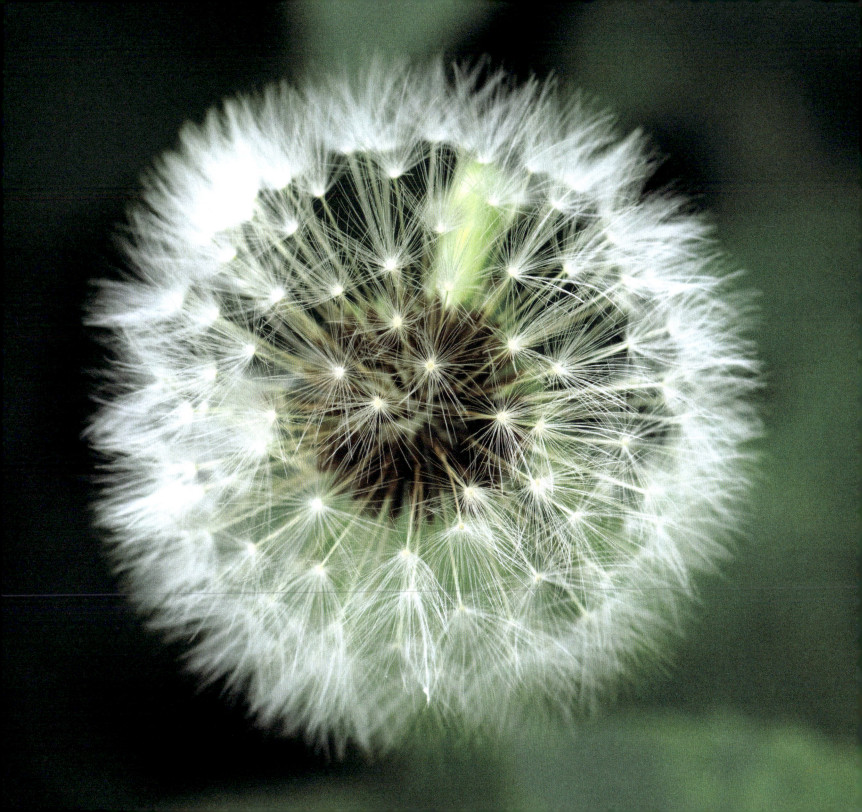

HERBAL MILK INFUSIONS OR DECOCTIONS

PERFECT FOR IMBOLC

Organic milks of various sorts may be used to make delicious botanically infused or decocted extracts by simply following the directions on p. 46 while replacing the water element with a milk.

These smooth milky beverages may be enjoyed either hot or cold, whichever is preferred, and are perfect for convalescence, being comforting, soothing *and* highly nutritious.

The richer in nourishing fats the milks are, the more likely they will be to draw out the lipid-based constituents of the botanicals being infused or decocted into them and to hold onto their wonderful imbrued flavours, making for an extraordinary taste experience that delights the senses.

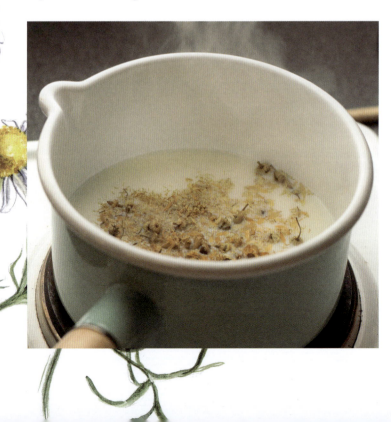

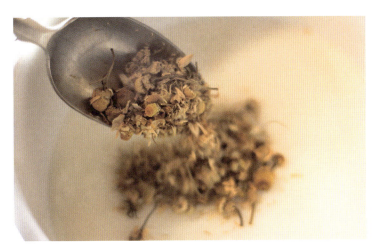

Oat milk offers a cooling and soothing alternative to dairy, as does soya, while the nut-based milks (e.g. hazelnut and almond) are sumptuously nourishing.

Chamomile milk, pictured here, is a lovely milk infusion to try at bedtime. To make this we simply infused a good, heaped teaspoon of the dried flowers in a mugful of warm milk. As before, a little honey may be added if required.

The naturally soporific effects of a warm milky drink may be therapeutically enhanced by the botanicals that are infused into it – dried chamomile flowers, hops, cowslip flowers, passionflower, valerian root, vervain, lime (*Linden*) flowers and lavender may all be tried, with a 'sleep time blend' being prepared from several. Warm milk has long been noted as being effectively sleep-inducing and this could in part be due to the high calcium and vitamin D content of the milk itself, as both of these compounds are believed to augment the body's natural production of melatonin – the 'night time hormone' intrinsically involved in the governance of our circadian rhythms and sleep.

Author's note: *If you wish to learn more about how to prepare tea blends effectively, please join one of our Herbology Fine Teas of the World short courses, which we run during the summer at the Royal Botanic Garden Edinburgh.*

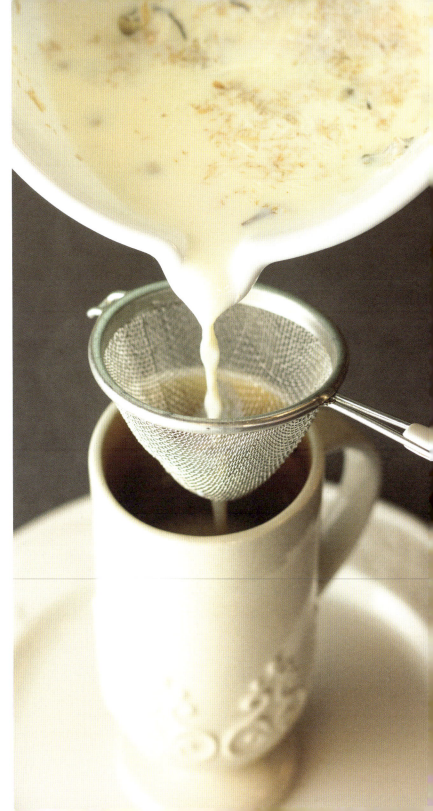

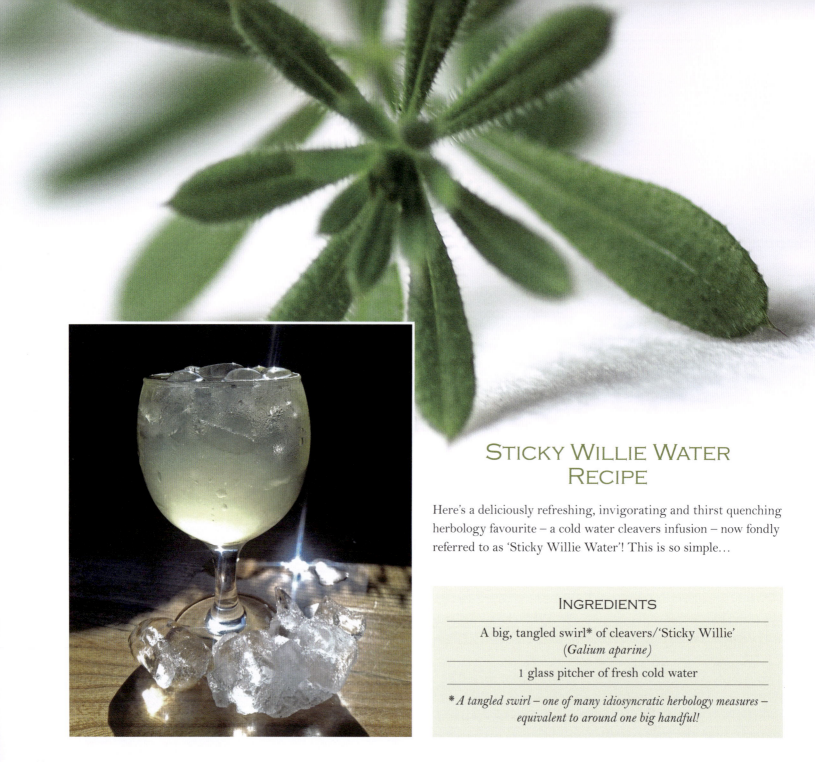

STICKY WILLIE WATER RECIPE

Here's a deliciously refreshing, invigorating and thirst quenching herbology favourite – a cold water cleavers infusion – now fondly referred to as 'Sticky Willie Water'! This is so simple…

INGREDIENTS

A big, tangled swirl* of cleavers/'Sticky Willie'
(*Galium aparine*)

1 glass pitcher of fresh cold water

* A tangled swirl – one of many idiosyncratic herbology measures – equivalent to around one big handful!

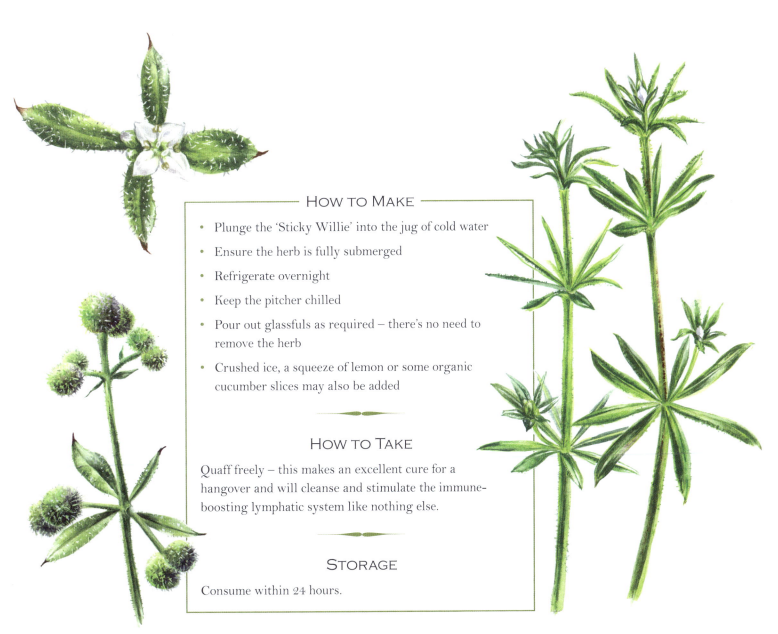

HOW TO MAKE

- Plunge the 'Sticky Willie' into the jug of cold water

- Ensure the herb is fully submerged

- Refrigerate overnight

- Keep the pitcher chilled

- Pour out glassfuls as required – there's no need to remove the herb

- Crushed ice, a squeeze of lemon or some organic cucumber slices may also be added

HOW TO TAKE

Quaff freely – this makes an excellent cure for a hangover and will cleanse and stimulate the immune-boosting lymphatic system like nothing else.

STORAGE

Consume within 24 hours.

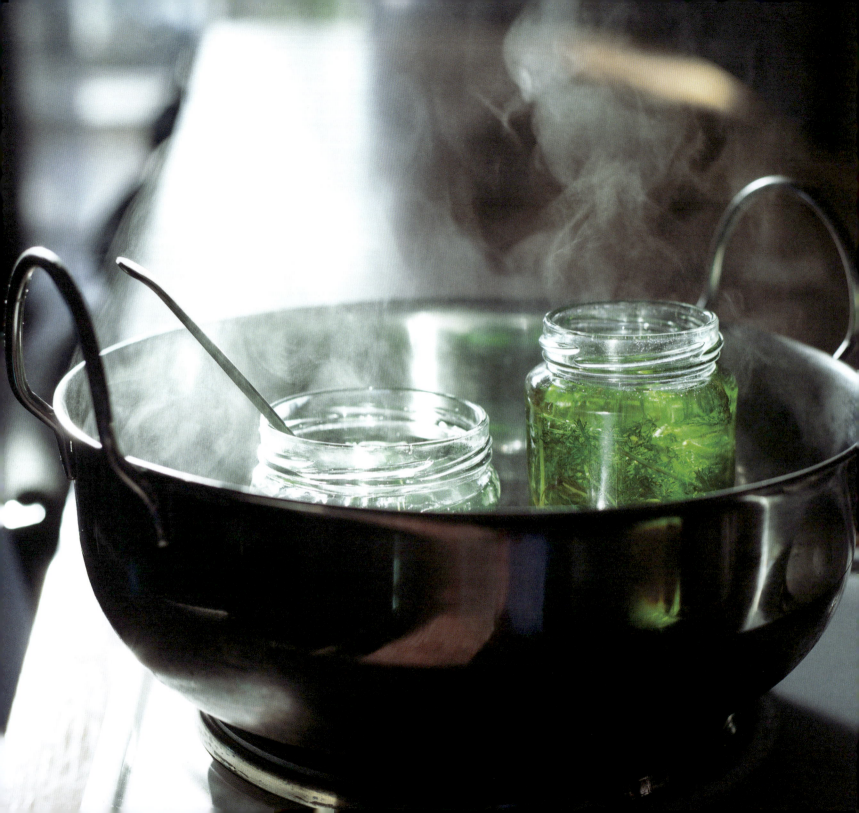

II.

GREEN HERB OINTMENTS & BOTANICAL INFUSED OILS

FIXED BASE OILS

Fixed base oils may be used to prepare luxuriant green herb–infused oils (the first step in our green herb ointment making), as well as being ingredients in many other topical remedies. Fixed base oils are generally the (vegetable) oils expressed from the crushed fruit or seed of a botanical – organic cold pressed oils are considered the best. Almond and olive oils are the most frequently used in herbal remedy making. Many of the fixed oils have a nourishing as well as therapeutic value.

However, by far the greatest use of fixed oils is to provide the base ingredient for herb-infused oils – lipid botanical jewels that they are! Herb-infused oils are made by infusing fresh or dried herbs in a cold pressed fixed base oil. This is a way to solubilise the therapeutic constituents of the herb so that they may be used topically in vulnerary formulations e.g. unguents, creams, lotions, liniments and pastes.

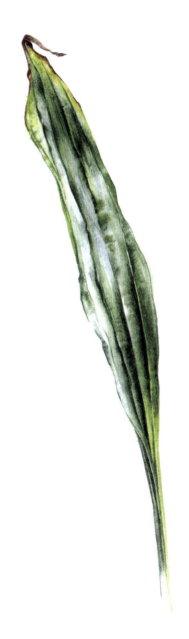

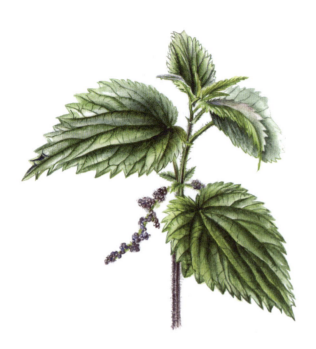

GREEN HERB-INFUSED OIL RECIPE

INGREDIENTS

Herb
(choose a vulnerary herb, p. 34)

Base oil
(a cold pressed olive oil – no dubious fats!)

Beeswax
(best sourced from a local beekeeper)

HOW TO MAKE

For cold infused oils (using fresh herbs):

- Allow the herbs to wilt overnight

- Place the herbs in a glass jar (until the jar is just over half full) and cover with base oil

- Lid the jar

- Store the jar in a cool dark place for a fortnight or so, ensuring the herbs remain submerged

- Shake the jar daily

- Once the oil has infused, strain out the herb

For hot infused oils (using dried herbs):

- Crush the dried herbs in a pestle and mortar until roughly ground

- Place the herbs in a jar in a bain-marie

- Add double the amount of fixed oil to herb

- Heat the oil gently for a couple of hours (ensure that the bain-marie doesn't simmer dry during this time)

- Remove the jar from the heat and strain out the herbs

HOW TO USE

Infused botanical oils have their own inherent therapeutic values and may be applied topically to the cutaneous tissues. Alternatively, with the addition of a little molten beeswax (or candelilla wax) and a few drops of essential oil, they may be transformed into a myriad of healing balms, ointments and unguents, to delight the senses and soothe mind, body and soul.

STORAGE

Infused oils may be stored in the fridge in lidded and labelled glass bottles or jars, and are best used within several months.

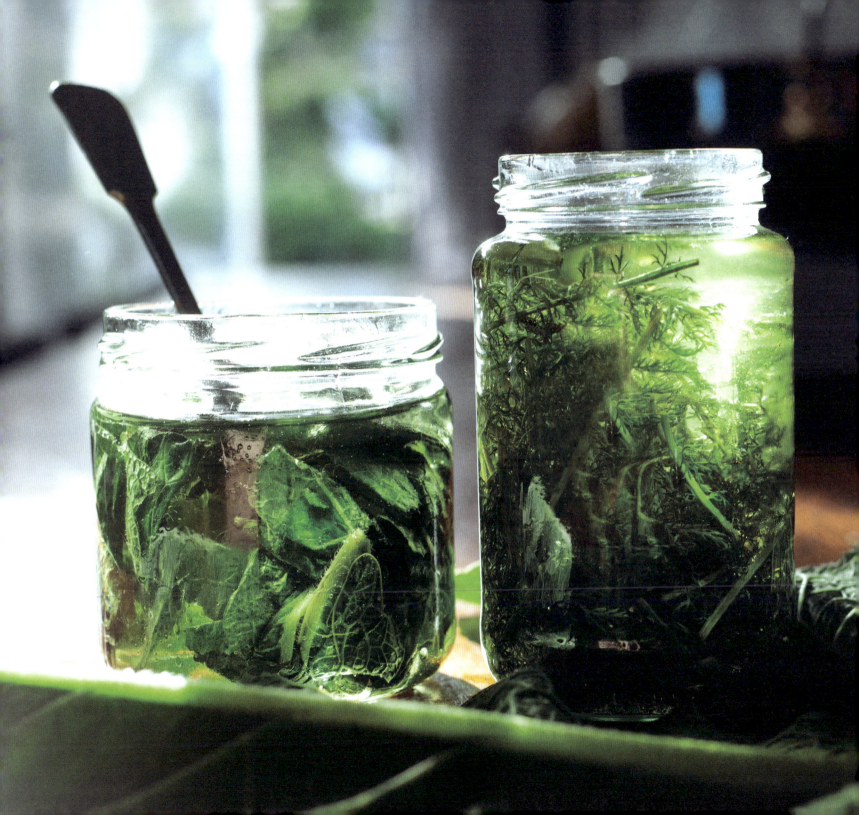

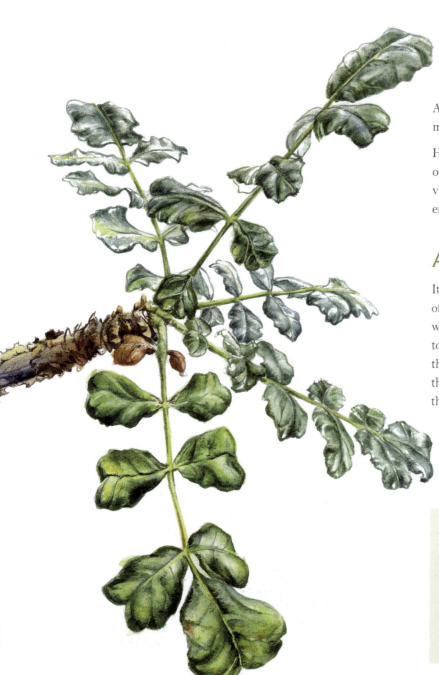

OINTMENTS

An ointment is an oil and wax-based remedy. It is traditionally made using a solution of herb-infused oil and molten beeswax.

Here's a very simple herbology recipe to follow to make your own green herb ointment. It is infinitely adaptable (see the list of vulnerary herbs, p. 34) and will yield an all-round sumptuously emollient remedy for slow to heal wounds.

A LITTLE OINTMENT FOLKLORE

It was believed that witches prepared their own particular form of unguents made from a blend of fat and psychotropic botanicals, which allegedly gave them the ability to fly high on their brooms to Sabbat celebrations – a concept that became a fearful one during the witch hunts, or so-called 'burning times', when it was rumoured that the fat of these ointments was rendered, most wickedly, from the murdered bodies of unbaptised babies!

GREEN HERB OINTMENT RECIPE

INGREDIENTS

1 handful of fresh green (vulnerary) herb

Half a jam jar of almond or other base oil

5 tsp of beeswax (per 100ml oil)

5–8 drops of a soothing, antiseptic or anti-inflammatory essential oil (e.g. lavender, tea tree, eucalyptus, frankincense)

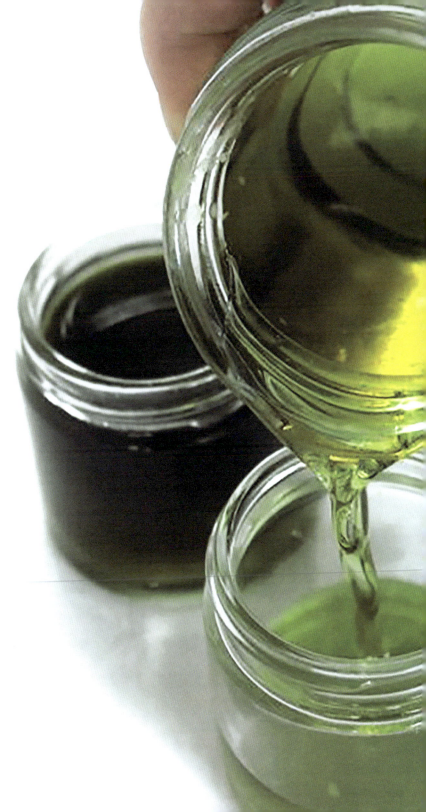

HOW TO MAKE

- Place the crushed herb in an empty, robust honey or jam jar and cover with oil

- Stand jar (with no lid) in a pan of warm water, creating a bain-marie

- Make sure that the water only reaches about halfway up the jar

- Gently heat the water and allow to simmer for 20 minutes (note: a metal teaspoon placed in the jar will help to prevent it cracking during this time)

- Strain out the herb and return the jar (with its now infused oil) to the bain-marie

- Melt in the beeswax

- Carefully remove the jar from the pan and allow the mixture to cool and solidify

- Once the ointment has formed, lid the jar and label

HOW TO USE

Apply small amounts as needed to unbroken, slow to heal wounds and irritated cutaneous tissues. For external use only.

STORAGE

Store in a cool dark place (e.g. a cupboard) and use within a year of preparation.

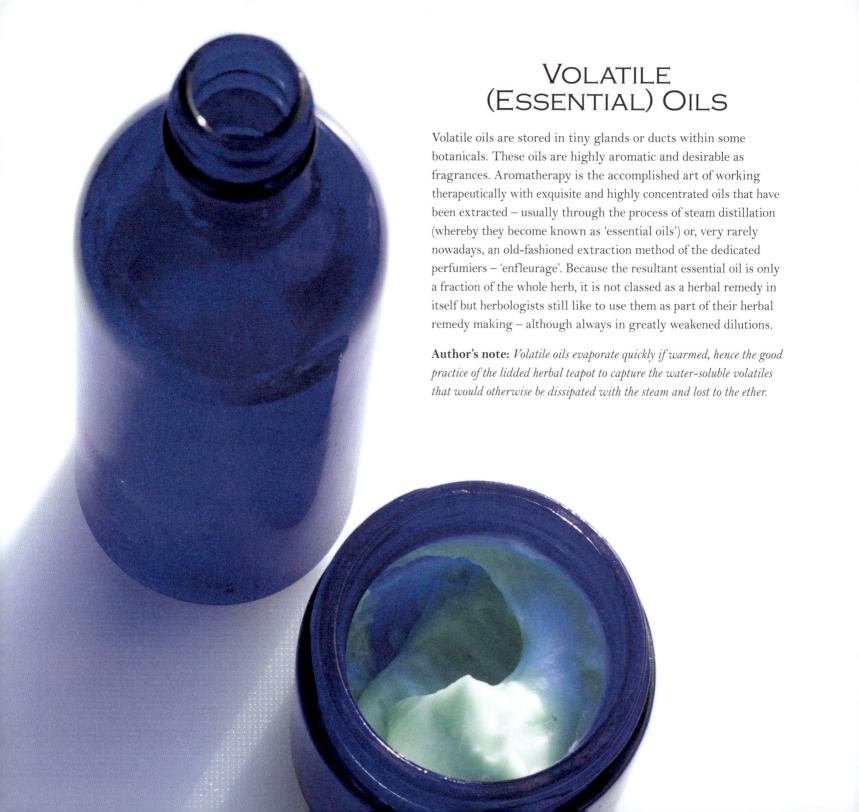

VOLATILE (ESSENTIAL) OILS

Volatile oils are stored in tiny glands or ducts within some botanicals. These oils are highly aromatic and desirable as fragrances. Aromatherapy is the accomplished art of working therapeutically with exquisite and highly concentrated oils that have been extracted – usually through the process of steam distillation (whereby they become known as 'essential oils') or, very rarely nowadays, an old-fashioned extraction method of the dedicated perfumiers – 'enfleurage'. Because the resultant essential oil is only a fraction of the whole herb, it is not classed as a herbal remedy in itself but herbologists still like to use them as part of their herbal remedy making – although always in greatly weakened dilutions.

Author's note: *Volatile oils evaporate quickly if warmed, hence the good practice of the lidded herbal teapot to capture the water-soluble volatiles that would otherwise be dissipated with the steam and lost to the ether.*

Blue Chamomile Balm Recipe

A very simple yet utterly delightful balm that makes the most of chamomile's blue-green azulene content and anti-inflammatory properties, inspired by the extraordinary azure blue of the pure essential oil ingredient.

Ingredients

50ml almond oil
3 tsp soft beeswax
8 drops of blue German chamomile essential oil

How to Make

- Warm the oil in a bain-marie
- Melt in the beeswax
- Once all the wax has liquefied, remove from the hob
- Add the essential oil drops
- Stir through thoroughly
- Pour into an ointment jar
- Allow to cool, lid and label

How to Use

Apply topically as needed to minor closed wounds and cutaneous irritations and to generally calm and soothe inflamed tissues.

Storage

Store in a cool dark place and use within a year of preparation.

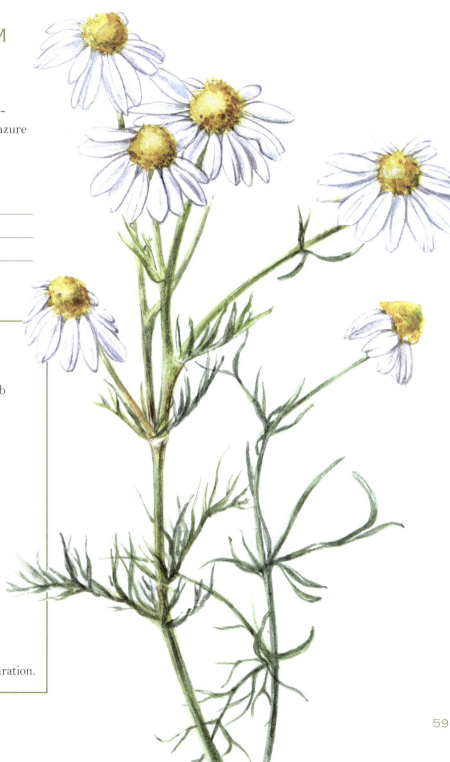

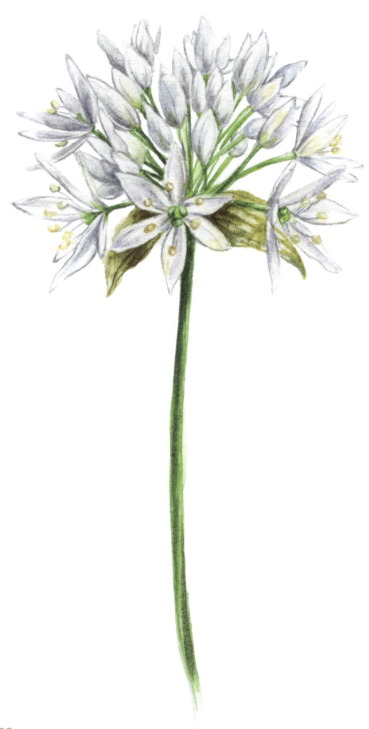

III.
REVITALISING VERNAL VINEGAR

Mineral-rich solutions of herb-infused organic apple cider vinegar are potent tonics, best enjoyed in the spring when they will help to revitalise, re-mineralise and rejuvenate the system after periods of winter hibernation. These ever-so-simple to prepare vinegar extracts hold their place within the 'nutraceutical' category of herbal formulation, being both highly medicinal and nutritional at the same time.

Enjoy the following recipe for its sheer exuberance of nutrient-rich spring greens and then perhaps experiment with one of the equally invigorating and intriguingly named 'Four Thieves Vinegars', which you will find among some of the older cookery books and herbals.

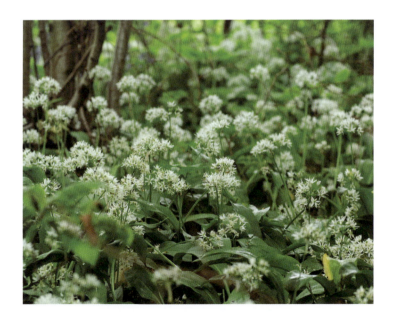

Green Herb Vinegar Recipe

Ingredients

1 cup (any size) organic apple cider vinegar, ideally with the 'mother'

½ cup fresh green rinsed and chopped nutritious herbs (e.g. nettle, dandelion, wild 'bear's' garlic)

Optional Ingredients
add to taste as preferred:

Chopped garlic cloves

Wild garlic 'bulbils' gathered after their flowers have bloomed

Red onion

Peppercorns

Fresh root (try small pieces of sweet cicely, ginger or horseradish)

Sprigs of tarragon, parsley, thyme etc.

Seeds (fennel, caraway, cardamom)

Black strapmolasses

Honey

How to Make

- Place the herbs in a sterilised glass jar
- Pour over the required amount of vinegar
- Add any other ingredients as preferred
- Lid and label the jar, and allow it to steep for at least a fortnight
- Shake occasionally
- Filter vinegar through unbleached coffee filter paper or cheesecloth
- Pour into a sterilised, decorative bottle

How to Take

Take up to three tablespoons neat or diluted in a little water as desired. Alternatively, work into a simple cold pressed olive oil, Dijon mustard and honey-based dressing and enjoy drizzled over other edible spring green herbs – delicious!

Storage

A herbal vinegar, stored in a cool dark place, will keep for over a year but as with all things, it is at its most potent when freshly made.

Author's note: *The 'mother' is a highly desirable and visible organism that may be found in unpasteurized (raw) vinegars. It is an organism that develops naturally on fermenting alcoholic liquids and helps turn apple cider into vinegar. Although the mother appears somewhat unattractive, it is harmless. The presence of the mother is indicative of a nutrient dense vinegar believed to be a probiotic that yields its own beneficial phenolic compounds.*

IV.
EASTER-LEDGE PUDDINGS

In northern rural parts of England it was a traditional spring practice to make a 'herb pudding'. These used to be prepared (and in some places still are) every year around Easter or during Lent, with the quintessential fresh green leaf ingredient of 'wester-ledges', more widely known as 'Easter-ledges' or bistort (*Bistorta officinalis*). Elsewhere referred to as 'Passion Pudding', these concoctions were highly valued as an easily affordable and supremely sustaining tonic food, full of vitamins, minerals and other nutrients. Below is the recipe for one such pudding that has become a fondly remembered 'remedy' from my own childhood; the making of which was an eagerly anticipated jollity of spring, when it could be found being 'brewed up' by my grandmother in a pink cottage high above the small hamlet of Thornthwaite in the Lake District. It is included here in loving memory of those happy times.

GREEN HERB PUDDING RECIPE

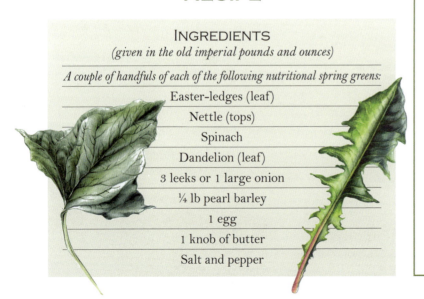

INGREDIENTS
(given in the old imperial pounds and ounces)

A couple of handfuls of each of the following nutritional spring greens:

Easter-ledges (leaf)
Nettle (tops)
Spinach
Dandelion (leaf)
3 leeks or 1 large onion
¼ lb pearl barley
1 egg
1 knob of butter
Salt and pepper

HOW TO MAKE

- Soak the barley into a bowl with 500ml (1 pint) of cold water overnight
- Put the barley and water into a heavy-bottomed pan
- Bring to the boil
- Simmer until barley is soft
- Add the herbs
- Simmer carefully altogether for about 30 minutes
- Drain well
- Spoon the mixture into a deep ovenproof pot
- Add the beaten egg and butter
- Bake for about 15 minutes at 180°C (355°F)
- Turn out onto a plate and season

HOW TO TAKE

Best enjoyed piping hot!

STORAGE

Best freshly made, the pudding can be stored for up to a week in the fridge.

Author's note: *Several big tablespoons of green herb vinegar (p. 61) could be added to taste before adding the egg and butter. Many recipes recommend that the herb pudding ingredients be steamed (tied up together in a muslin bag) rather than boiled and it may not be necessary for a pudding to be baked at the end.*

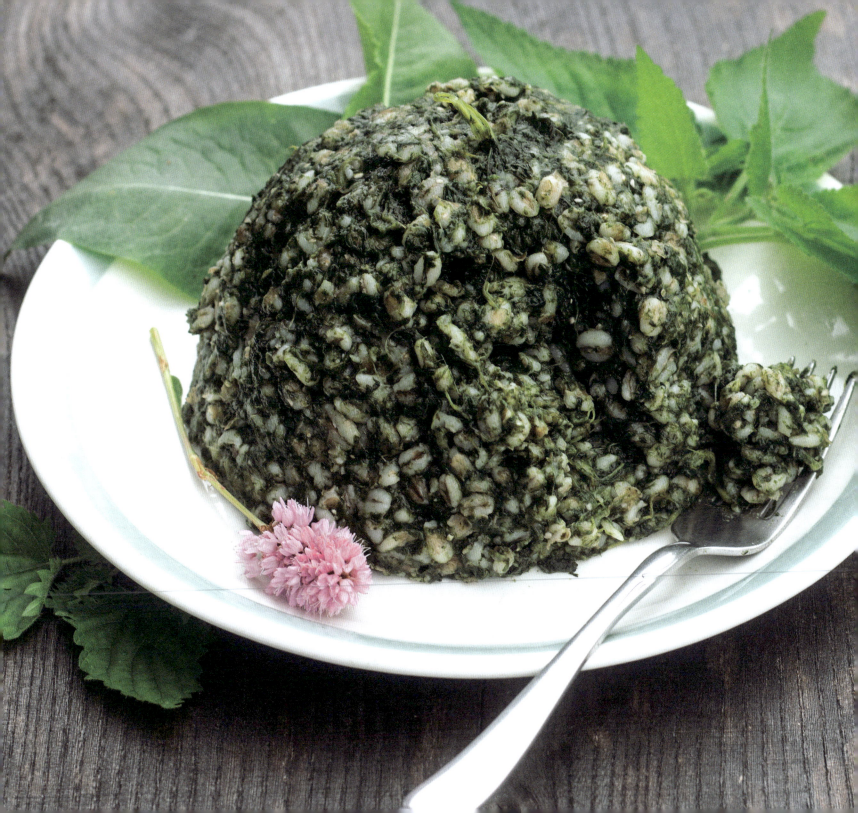

V.
WILLOW MILK BATH POWDERS

A NOTE ON IMBOLC

Willow is, as Culpeper tells us in his 17th century herbal *The English Physitian* (1652), under the influence of the moon, and as such is associated with all things feminine, intuitive and the element of water. One of the sacred trees of the Druids, it is intimately connected to Imbolc, a pagan festival of the Celtic tradition that marks the halfway point between the winter solstice and the spring equinox. It was known as the 'quickening time', when the first buds and lambs would appear and sap and milk would begin to flow.

There is nothing quite so soothing as a willow milk bath and the quintessential component of this recipe is the powdered willow itself, a perfect bath powder ingredient as the salicin compounds it holds are infinitely water soluble – rather like bathing in liquid aspirins!

Author's note: *Please don't be tempted to gather willow bark from trees in the wild – such a precious ingredient needs to be bought from a reputable herbal dispensary where you know it has been sustainably and responsibly sourced.*

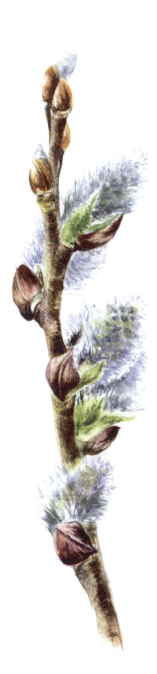

Willow Milk Bath Powder Recipe

Ingredients

3 heaped tsp of white willow bark (very finely powdered)

3 tbsp of milk powder (or finely powdered oats)

Optional: 5–8 drops of wintergreen essential oil

How to Make

- Measure the milk or oat powder into a bowl

- Add the powdered willow bark

- Mix the ingredients together

- Add the essential oil drops and stir through thoroughly

- Spoon the powder into soft muslin bags or squares and tie securely

How to Use

Place the muslin bag in a warm bath, squeeze the bag gently several times to help infuse the water, relax and enjoy!

Storage

Stored in a lidded pot or jar, this powdered formula will keep for several months.

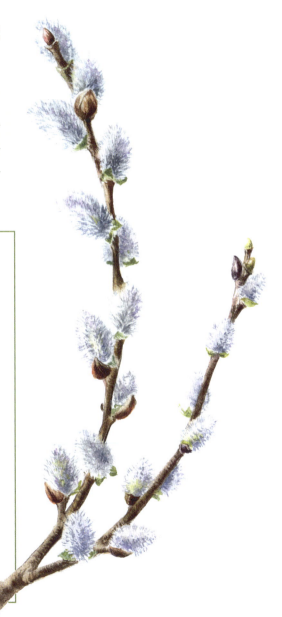

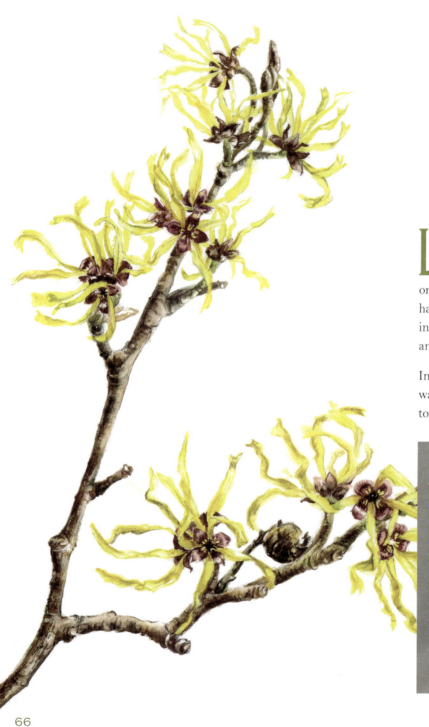

VI.
LOTIONS

Lotions are refreshingly light and gentle liquid formulations. There are innumerable recipes but witch hazel water lotion is one of the simplest of formulations to make, originally inspired by the joyful winter blooming Chinese witch hazel (*Hamamelis mollis*). It makes an excellent yet simple base, into which other herbal waters or distillates (in equal measure) and/or alcoholic extracts (in half measures) may be added.

In the following recipe, the alcoholic extracts of witch hazel water impart a cooling, mildly antiseptic and cleansing property to the lotion, while glycerine adds hydration.

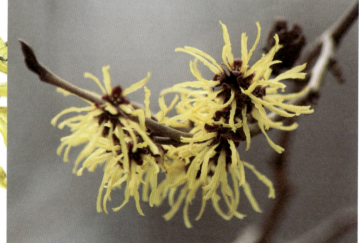

WITCH HAZEL WATER LOTION RECIPE

To help tone, refresh and hydrate the cutaneous tissues after winter's repose.

INGREDIENTS

3 parts witch hazel water (e.g. 300ml)

1½ parts glycerine (e.g. 150ml)

10 drops of citrus (e.g. grapefruit, lemon or lime) essential oil (use 1 drop per 40ml liquid)

HOW TO MAKE

- Pour the ingredients into a bottle
- Lid and label the bottle securely

HOW TO USE

External use only. Shake well before use – apply after bathing, body brushing or gentle exfoliation.

STORAGE

Store somewhere cool and dark for up to a year.

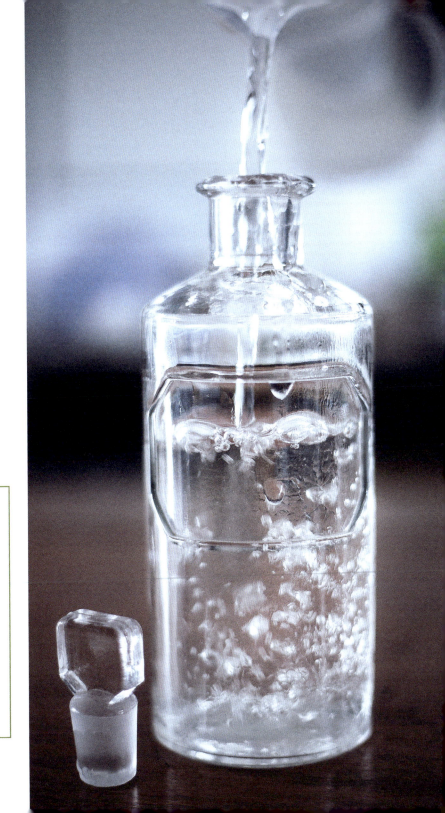

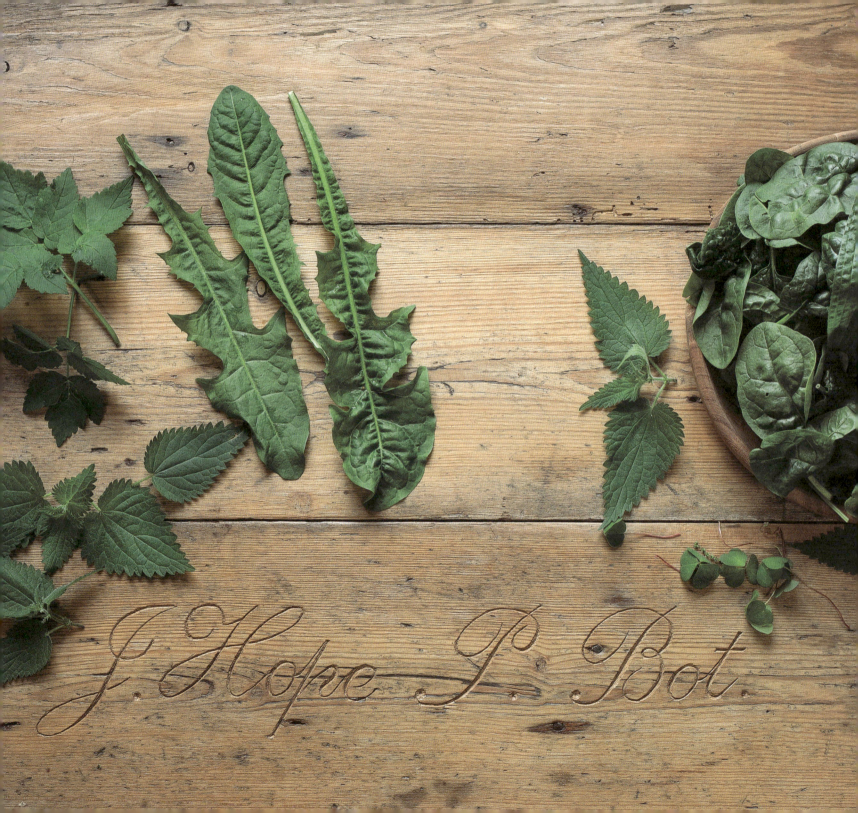

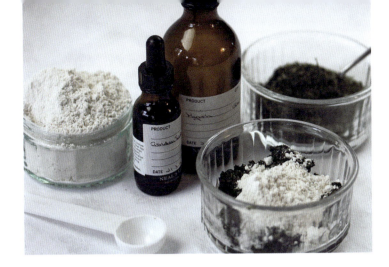

VII.

POULTICE POWDERS, PLASTERS & PASTES

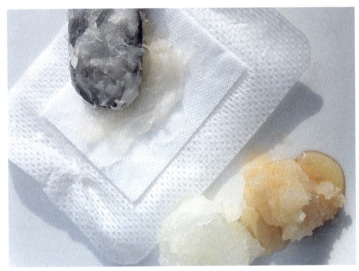

These three very traditional (topical) wound-healing herbal formulations are most easily differentiated by their nature and how they are prepared.

- A POULTICE is a simple herbal pad or wrap

- A PLASTER is a medicated herbal bandage made using a solution of waxes and oils into which herbal compounds may have been added

- A PASTE is a soft, pulped herbal formulation that may be smoothed directly onto the integument, or used in the preparation of a poultice

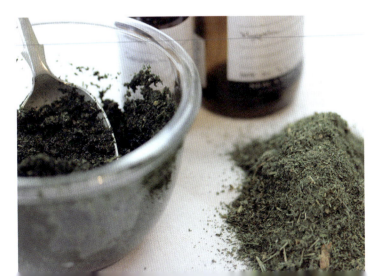

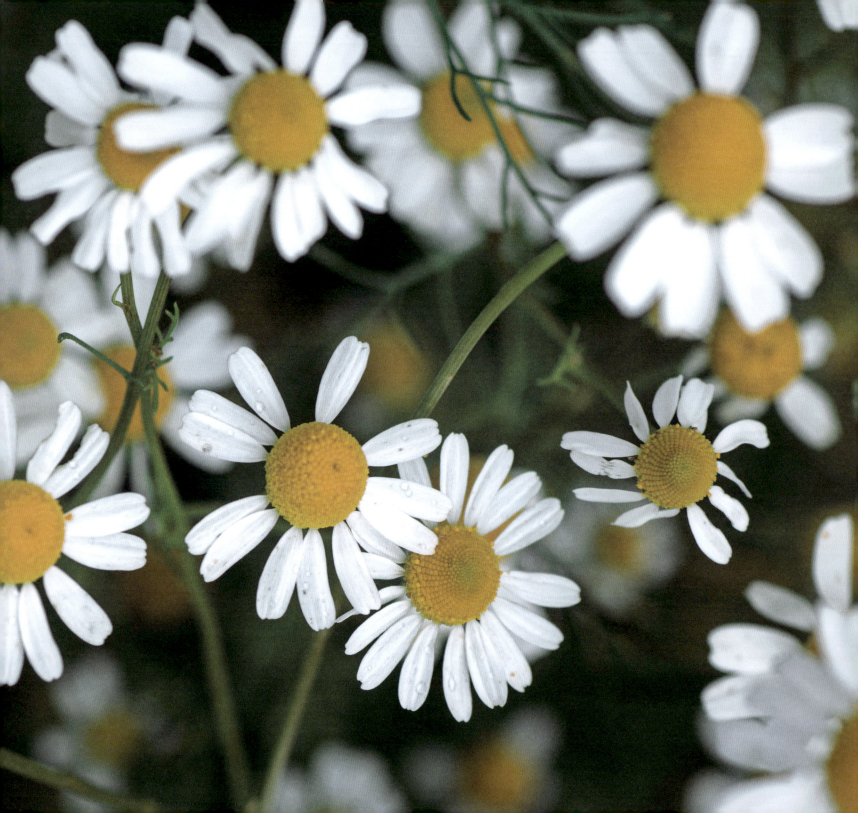

POULTICE (POWDERS)

A poultice is usually made by enclosing soft, semi-pulped or paste-like herbal ingredients (which may be most conveniently stored as ready-to-use dried powdered mixtures) that have been mixed with either water, honey or other healing fluids. Some appropriate herbs to try in the form of a poultice are noted on pp. 34–37. Poultices are generally used for imparting heat, although they may also be used for their refrigerant properties, to cool and even chill the integument when they are applied cold. The thermal effect of a poultice (whether hot or cold) is intended to enhance the therapeutic action of the compounds that they hold, which also aids their release of moisture to the body. Poultices may act as a local stimulant or relaxant as required.

PIPING HOT POULTICES (HANDLE WITH CARE!)

If a poultice is required to impart heat (which can be extremely comforting), it needs to be applied to the body as hot as possible – but not so hot that it scalds or burns the underlying integument! Keep the poultice moist and warm by placing a waterproof wrap over it and periodically replenish the herbal ingredients to reinvigorate the remedy.

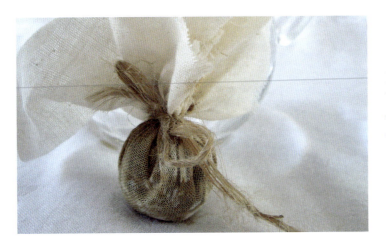

DRIED OR FRESH HERBS?

Dried poultice powders (a mixture of dried and powdered vulnerary herbs) are wonderful things to have readily to hand in a herbal first aid box and may be stored in a cool, dry place for up to a year in small airtight tins or packages. In the past, powders of this sort were often used directly on cleansed and superficial wounds in the form of healing dusting agents. Recently there has been a resurgence of interest in the possible applications of these old wound-healing herbal powders, as they are made up of purely natural ingredients with absorptive, aromatic, antiseptic and anti-inflammatory synergistic properties. A contemporary homeopathic recipe (prepared in India) for a natural wound care powder uses extracts of calendula and arnica, in a powder base of wild field mint and sandalwood. That said, for home herbal use, one may choose either dried or fresh herbs to make a poultice. If dried herbs are used they should always be ground to a soft powder, with just enough liquid added to make a thick paste. If fresh green leaves are used, simply heat, bruise and break them up finely. It may be appropriate to apply fresh green herbs to the affected parts directly, e.g. a dock leaf to a nettle sting.

A 'DRAWING' POULTICE

Poultices are excellent for inflamed glandular nodes and 'eruptions'– such as a boil, carbuncle or an abscess. A simple drawing (sometimes more descriptively referred to as a 'ripening' or suppuration) poultice may be made as follows: prepare a soft composition with slippery elm powder (a more sustainable alternative would be hot mashed potato) and warm water, adding a quantity of crushed raw or boiled onion, or hot moist bread. Powdered earth clays (lubricated to a paste) may also be used in this way (e.g. a kaolin poultice).

PLASTERS

Plasters (or 'emplastra' as they were formerly known) were a way of ensuring that herbal ingredients remained against the integument for a therapeutically optimum amount of time. The old *Edinburgh Pharmacopoeia* (1699) is a rich source of early emplastra recipes, including what may well have been the very soothing anodyne plaster, *Emplastrum anodinum*, mingled discreetly among the rather less appealing blistering plaster, *Emplastrum epispasticum*, and our personal favourite: a 'plaster of frogs with mercury'!

The plaster itself is a paste-like substance and was generally made from herbal ingredients mixed into a soft resin, lanolin or molten beeswax. It was semi-solid until gently warmed in a bain-marie, when it would liquefy sufficiently to be spread on a suitable piece of gauze, muslin or bandage. In the past, the malleable plaster formulation was smoothed out and evenly distributed with a bespoke heated iron and the plasters were applied warm.

Here's a traditional plaster-base formulation. Except for beeswax, the following ingredients (once in regular therapeutic usage) are less frequently encountered in herbal remedies nowadays and some may even be considered inappropriate by the contemporary herbologist! This rather charming old practice can be easily adapted to create a lubricating, comforting emollient unguent as demonstrated (right).

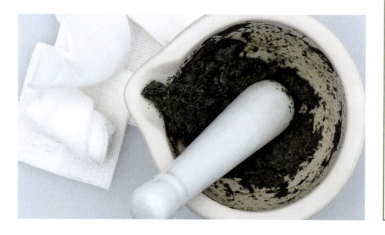

A TRADITIONAL PLASTER-BASE RECIPE

INGREDIENTS

100g beeswax
50ml castor oil
50g anhydrous lanolin
200g soft paraffin

Author's note: *Finely powdered herbs may be added to the plaster base: use one part herb to four parts base. A fluid extract of up to 20%, or vulnerary essential oil (5 drops to every 50g of base) can be used instead of powdered herbs.*

HOW TO MAKE

- Melt all the ingredients together in a bain-marie
- Stir well to mix thoroughly
- Keep stirring as the mixture cools, and when tepid, spread on as wide a bandage as required

This base may then be perfused with vulnerary herbs in their powdered, liquid or distilled extract form. For a non-oily plaster a glycerine-gel base may be used. Simply melt the gel base in a bain-marie and add appropriate alcoholic fluid extracts. Stir to mix well and then, just before it solidifies, dip the bandage into the mixture.

HOW TO USE

Apply warm to closed and slow-to-heal wounds.

STORAGE

Store all plasters between waxed papers in a fridge. Use within one month or store indefinitely frozen.

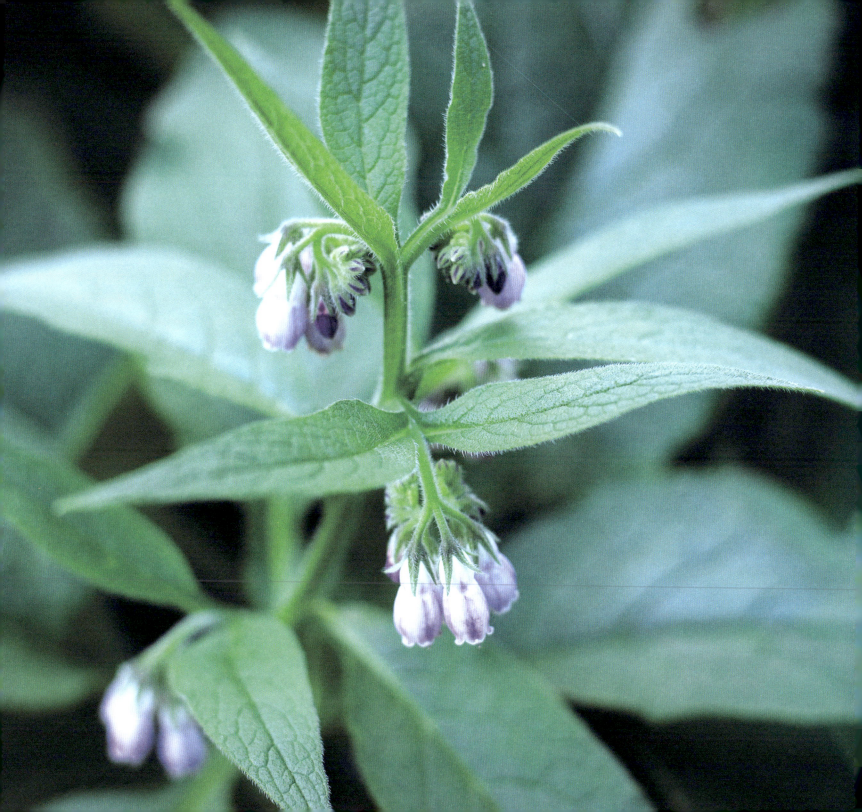

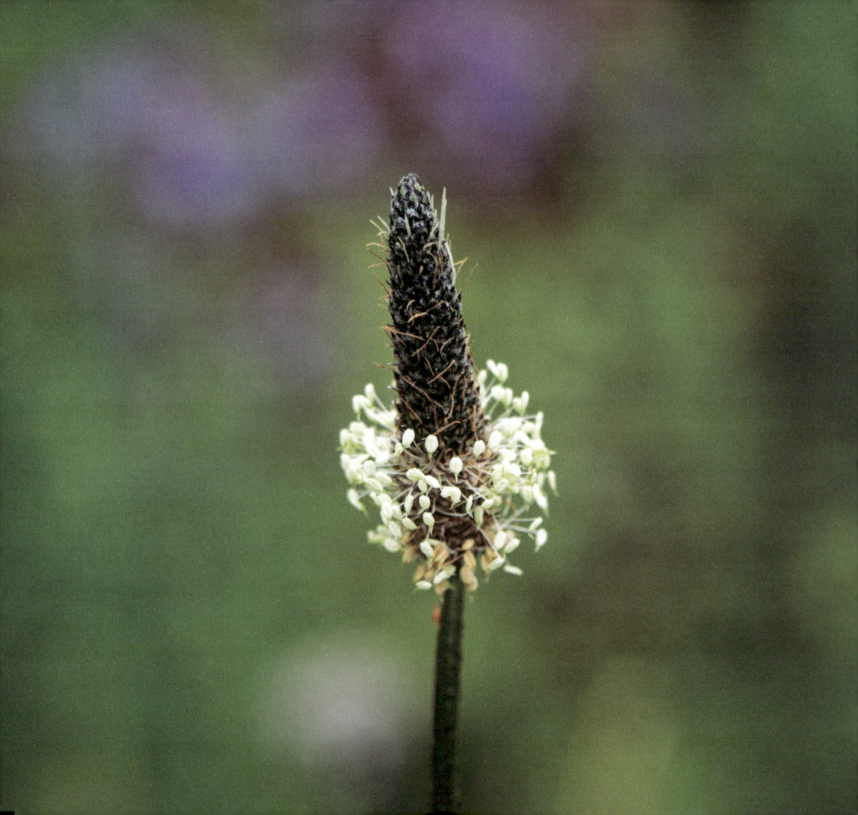

PASTES

For herbology purposes we tend to consider pastes purely as another form of a topical vulnerary, wound-healing remedy. In the past, however, they were equally valued as potential oral formulations and from the more contemporary and culinary side of things, recipes for fresh, soft-leaved herbal pastes are quite the thing for anyone wanting to preserve tender nutritious greens, while sugared pulped fruit provides another possibility for a most delicious paste.

For a topical vulnerary paste such as the one overleaf, any of the wound-healing herbs (pp. 34–37) may be used.

Generally, vulnerary pastes are made from dried herbs ground to the softest, finest powders. However, pulped fresh herbs may also be used as a form of paste. If you are using fresh green herbs it is often sufficient simply to crush these until the juice released achieves the desired consistency of the paste you are after. Generally, pastes are best made up as 'simples' i.e. using only one herbal ingredient at a time.

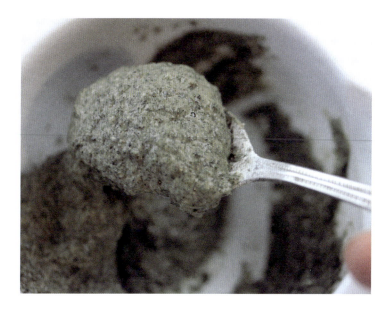

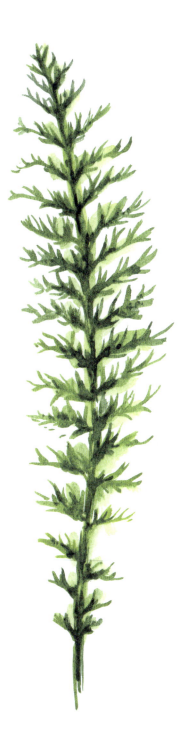

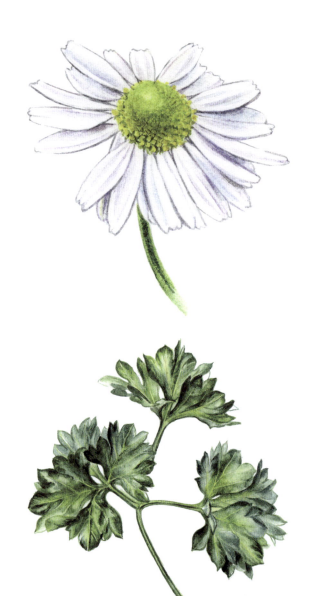

EDIBLE PULP PASTE RECIPE

INGREDIENTS

1 handful of fresh, soft green, edible herb
such as parsley

HOW TO MAKE

- Add a small amount of cold water to the herb (or a little parsley infusion for a double hit!)
- Gently blend to a pulp-like consistency

HOW TO TAKE

Mix into homemade sauces or spring soups.

STORAGE

Use freshly made or freeze small amounts in ice cube trays until required.

Author's note: *This recipe is not suitable for the hard, woodier-stemmed herbs – use soft tender greens only!*

Topical Vulnerary Paste
Recipe

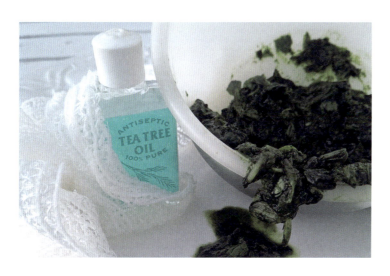

Ingredients

Fresh herbs to try:

Plantain (leaf)

Yarrow (leaf)

Bogbean (*Menyanthes trifoliata*) (leaf)

Dried herbs to try:

Powdered chamomile (flower)

Finely powdered oats

Powdered marshmallow (leaf and root in equal parts)

How to Make

- Add a little cold water to your dried herbs (or even better, a vulnerary herbal infusion) or pulp fresh herbs
- Work the mixture into a paste
- Optional: add some local honey or vulnerary herb-infused oil

How to Use

Smooth a deep layer of herbal paste onto the body where needed, cover with gauze and/or a waterproof dressing and secure with a bandage. After several hours, remove the wrappings and rinse the used remedy away. You can re-apply fresh herbal paste if necessary.

Storage

Green herbal pastes need to be refrigerated and should be used within one week of preparation, although they may be stored frozen for up to a year. If the herbs used are dried, and especially if honey is included as an ingredient, then the remedy will store without refrigeration for several weeks.

Author's note: *Excellent oils for vulnerary pastes are the more restorative and nourishing botanical oils intended for topical use such as sea buckthorn, rosehip and argan oil.*

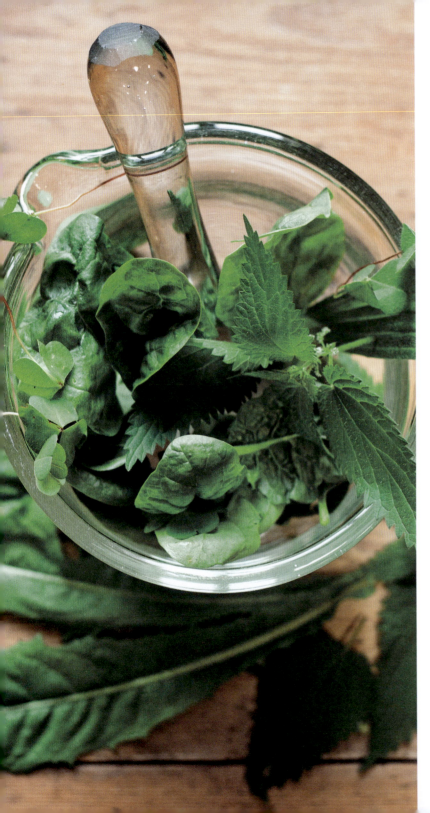

VIII.
JUICES (*SUCCI*)

In the 17th century the word 'juice' (especially in reference to a medicinal liquid) would carry a somewhat different connotation than it does today, being more likely to refer to an aqueous extract like a decoction, rather than an expression of botanical saps and fluids. The *Edinburgh Pharmacopoeia* (1699) notes only one such juice, *Succus glycyrrhizae*, known as juice of liquorice, which was brought by sea from distant shores (usually Spain) and about which we know very little – except that it probably more closely resembled a liquorice water than our contemporary understanding of a 'juice'.

Herbology's favourite wild forager, Monica Wilde, has shared her recollections of a very memorable form of liquorice juice brought into herbal dispensaries as big sticky gooey blocks of solid extract that would then be melted down and used as an ingredient in lozenges and cough mixtures etc. Another earlier herbal (*Herbal Simples Approved for Modern Uses of Cure* (1897) by Dr William Thomas Fernie) describes small phials of water with bits of this 'Spanish juice' being shaken to make a solution that increased in value the darker and thicker it became.

A relatively recently concocted herbology juice, created as part of our green pharmacy at Royal Botanic Garden Edinburgh, takes the more familiar form of a blend of several individually expressed juices from a variety of soft and succulent green botanicals and orchard fruits – feel free to add your own juice of liquorice if you wish!

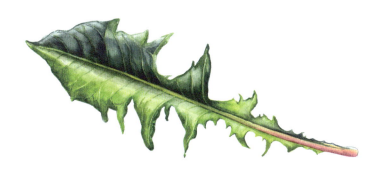
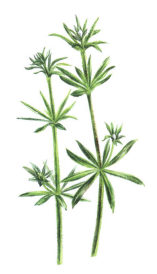
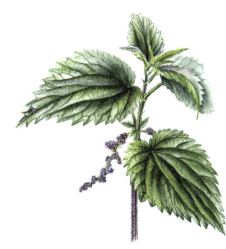

GREEN HERB JUICE RECIPE

INGREDIENTS

A couple of generous handfuls of mixed fresh green herbs

1 squeeze of organic lemon juice

1 tsp fresh ginger root

300ml fresh organic apple or pear juice

FRESH GREEN HERBS TO TRY

Organic spinach is the perfect 'green' to yield the bulk of your juice extract, and it juices so readily! Any of the following 'wild weeds' will add their own character to the juice blend, so sample small amounts of each to see which you prefer. Use tender leaf only and be mindful of dandelion's 'piss en lit' reputation!

- CLEAVERS (*Galium aparine*)
- DANDELION (*Taraxacum officinale*)
- CHICKWEED (*Stellaria media*)
- SPRING BEAUTY (*Claytonia perfoliata*)
- WILD 'BEAR'S' GARLIC (*Allium ursinum*)
- NETTLE (*Urtica dioica*)

HOW TO MAKE

- Gather your herbs
- Rinse the herbs in cold water
- Grate the ginger root
- Add the herb and ginger root to the juicer (an old-fashioned hand-cranked juicer is ideal for this recipe)
- Juice until around 20-30ml of liquid is extracted
- Add the extracted herbal and ginger juice to apple or pear juice
- Add the lemon juice and stir all the juices together

HOW TO USE

Once prepared, share with a friend and enjoy straight away!

STORAGE

Fresh juice extracts will keep for one day if refrigerated and may be frozen for later use.

IX.
BELTANE FLOWER CORDIAL

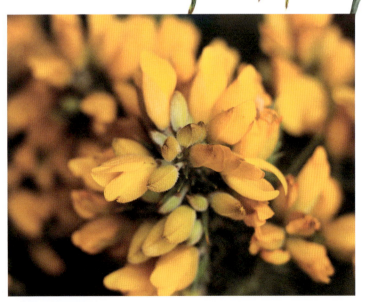

Every year in the UK, as the sun sets on the 30 April, Beltane may be witnessed taking place. Faithful re-enactments of this ancient pagan fire festival are quite something to behold, and in Edinburgh especially the only place to be on such a night is amidst the thronging crowd on Carlton Hill, where a torchlit yet dusky procession of masked and curiously adorned characters play out their respective roles in this ancient celebration of the rites of spring. Their dances, evocations and drummings have reached far into the starlit nights of many years and seemingly carry the spirit of Celtic souls through a transitional journey from the colder darkness of winter towards the warmer light of summer.

In recognition of this time (around 1 May), a very particular 'solution sweet' – a golden gorse flower cordial – is recommended. It is truly delicious.

Beltane Flower Cordial Recipe

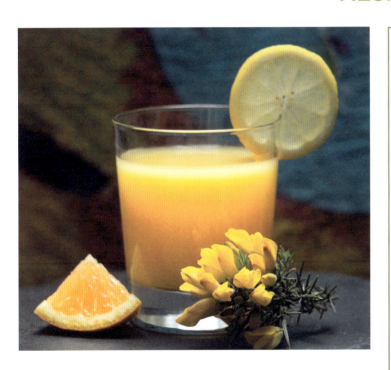

How to Make

- Dissolve the sugar and the water together in a big pan
- Gently bring the syrupy mixture to the boil
- Boil rapidly for 7 minutes
- Remove from the hob and add the rest of the ingredients
- Allow to steep (infuse) for 5 minutes or so
- Strain through muslin, a fine gauge sieve, or clean cotton handkerchief
- Bottle and label with the date of preparation

How to Take

Take three to five teaspoons neat as a healing syrup, or dilute with chilled water and ice to yield a refreshing and soothing summer cordial – the latter may be drunk freely.

Storage

Keep refrigerated and use within a couple of weeks of preparation. Alternatively, pour the syrup into appropriate receptacles and freeze so that it might be enjoyed even in the depths of winter!

Ingredients

A couple of big handfuls of gorse flowers

21 fl. oz water

8oz raw cane caster sugar

Zest of 1 orange

Juice of 1 lemon

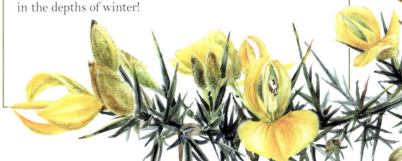

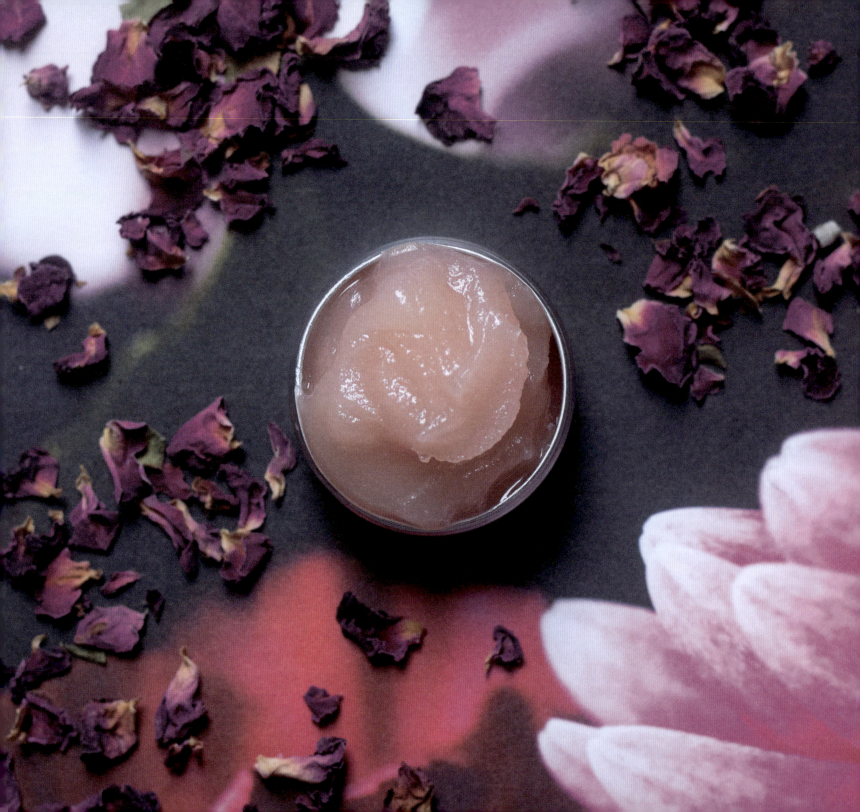

An Extract from Edinburgh Pharmacopoeia (1699)

An Original Ointment Recipe

As you have been introduced (in some detail!) to simple ointment making in this chapter and given this remedy's various manifestations among the ensuing recipes throughout this book, we thought it apt to include an ointment recipe here as our *Pharmacopoeia* extract of choice for spring.

The most benign ointment recipe from those listed in the *Edinburgh Pharmacopoeia* (1699) is the *Unguentum Rosacuum, Vulgo Pomantum*, more commonly known as a pomatum or rose ointment (oil of rhodium):

> 'Take any quantity of Hog's lard, cut it into small pieces, put it into a glazed earthen vessel, and pour thereon as much spring water as will float some inches above it: Let them stand together for ten days, the water being shifted once a day, then melt the lard, with a very soft heat, and throw it into a sufficient quantity of Rose-Water; wherein let it well worke'd; then pouring the water off from it, add a few drops of Oil of Rhodium.'

Ointments, *unguenta*, are recorded in the the *Edinburgh Pharmacopoeia* with oil, hog's lard or goat's suet used as a base for the healing herbs along with either a white or yellow wax (beeswax) ingredient. Other far more dubious ingredients within these formulations included quicksilver (mercury); chemical compounds like spirit of nitre (ethyl nitrite spirit), spermaceti (a waxy lubricating liquid sourced from whales) and the familiar calamine (essentially zinc and iron oxides in a phenolic or limewater solution); minerals including litharge of gold (which consists of lead oxide mixed with red lead), powdered blister beetles, *Cantharides* (once thought to be an aphrodisiac) and white lead, *Ceruse*, used as a pigment to create the white ointment, *Unguentum album*, noted in the *Pharmacopoeia*. Venice turpentine, distilled from the oleoresin of the larch tree, *Larix decidua*, appears to have been a fairly frequently used ingredient in ointments of this time. A variety of what would nowadays be regarded as well-chosen herbs are recorded in the receipts, for example, *Unguentum Vermifugum* includes wormwood, rose ointment, rose water and an ointment for burns, *Unguentum ambusta* references the elder – although the use of the leaves of henbane and hemlock and deadly nightshade berries are also to be found among the ingredients of other ointments.

Author's note: *This notorious Materia medica is not for the faint-hearted and definitely not for us – please do not try at home!*

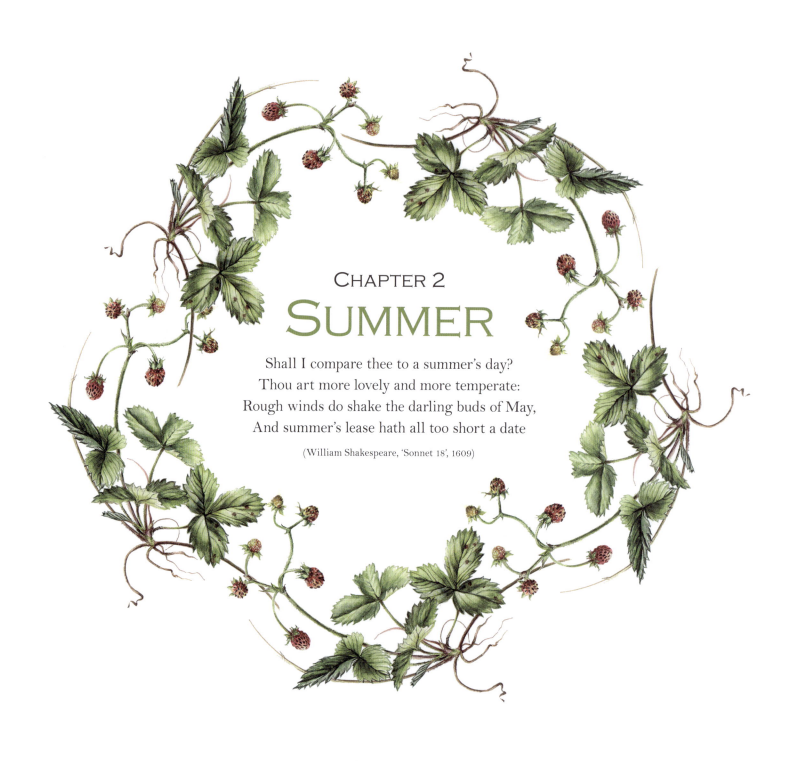

CHAPTER 2
SUMMER

Shall I compare thee to a summer's day?
Thou art more lovely and more temperate:
Rough winds do shake the darling buds of May,
And summer's lease hath all too short a date

(William Shakespeare, 'Sonnet 18', 1609)

We are almost unaware of that first true sense of summer when it comes – borne to us as it so often is on an unexpectedly refreshing intake of cool and fragrant morning air or heralded by the sound of a stirring bumblebee droning sleepily around awakening floral borders.

Summer then is upon us and we may breathe it in deeply at last – all the dreams that it holds and its distant hazy promises of blissfully perfect days that seem to stretch ahead of us forever as if they will never end.

How eagerly we may embrace the most pleasurable of our green-fingered pursuits at this time, including the carefree musings in and around our own or friends' beloved gardens. Indeed, whenever the working hours are done or simply abandoned, we make good our escape. Perhaps heading as far as the coast, tantalised by the sea's shimmering, sparkling light and on to where we might indulge in the sun-kissed satisfactions of lazy days – such are the joys of an alfresco summer life!

At this time of year in the northern hemispheres it never quite grows dark and the twilight hours that bookend our days seem to meld into one in an otherworldly half-light that exists somewhere between the hours that fall after dusk and extend until just before the dawn – the nocturnal creatures' realm. These are the nights around midsummer that feel almost intoxicating, enfolded in a soft warmth, fragranced with blossoms and studded with stars.

Then at the height of it all, the Celtic fire festival of Lughnasa flares into the heavens of late August, rejoicing in the gathering of bountiful crops and all of nature's many munificent blessings, as the resplendent gleaming orb of the harvest full moon rises low over the wheat fields.

It is on such nights as these if our location is conducive that we might realise the immortality of our own souls, standing before this magnificent moon much as our ancestors would have done. It's possible to become aware of our infinite connections to all elements of the natural world – from the tiniest stone, creature or flower to the deepest rhythms of the earth itself. To know that we too gaze out into the same eternal vastness of the Milky Way as our distant forefathers, following the celestial dust trails of the Perseids meteor showers across the starry wastes and other such legacies of a billion years.

Ah summer, if only we could hold on to it forever…

PHYSIC GARDEN DIARY

THINGS TO DO IN THE PHYSIC GARDEN

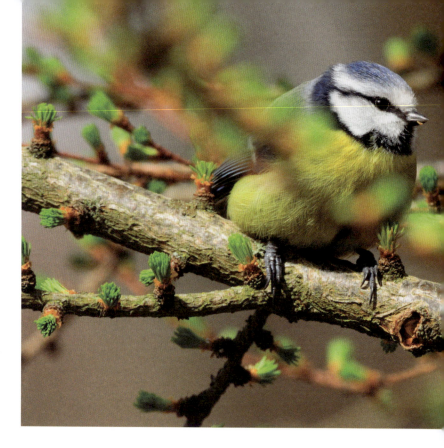

As the light extends and true warmth returns to the earth, the summertime quite literally extends the tasks and nurturing duties entailed for the diligent gardener. The ensuing months will bring some of the most beautiful blooms to bear and equally some of the most delightful fragrances. These are happy times in which a gardener may take the greatest of pleasure and pride in tending even the smallest collection of botanicals, witnessing the culmination of earlier labours coming to fruition.

Evelyn, in his *Kalendarium Hortense*, suggests sowing hot aromatic herbs and plants and advises: 'Ply the laboratory, and distill plants for waters, spirits.'

Evelyn also informs us that now is the time to nurture melons and bring oranges 'boldly out of the conservatory', while the honeybees in their hives may at last be granted their 'full liberty'.

We are not fortunate enough to be able to tend melons in our northern hemisphere herb beds, nor oranges for that matter. Instead, we turn our attention to a small selection of medicinal native soft fruits, such as blackcurrants and raspberries, and any bees (always welcome visitors) arrive at their pleasure from the neighbouring gardens.

As the eagerly awaited strawberry full moon approaches, the Garden's herbologists have compiled a list of things to do in June based on Evelyn's directions:

I.   Gather herbs in full. Evelyn notes: 'To keep dry; they keep and retain their virtue and sweet smell, better dry'd in the shade than the sun, whatever some pretend' – an astute observance that most herbalists would agree with

II. Gather snails after rain – a prudent and very benign (for the snails) piece of advice

III. Gather ripe flower seeds, at least those 'worth the saving'

IV. Befriend the birds in your garden. As Evelyn explains: 'For now the birds do grow sick of their feathers; therefore assist them with emulsions of the cooler seeds bruis'd in their water, as melons, cucumbers etc. Also give them succory, beets, groundsel, chick weed, fresh-gravel, and earth'

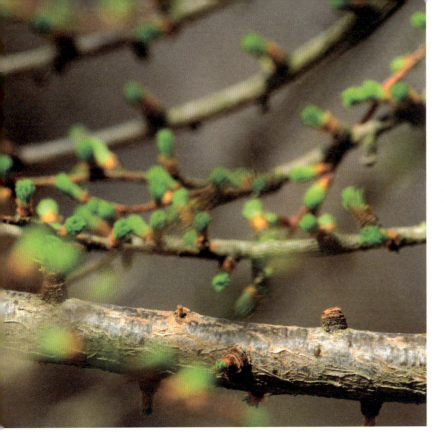

In August Evelyn advises:

X.   Deadhead roses

XI.   Pull up ripe onions and garlic

XII.   Gather seeds

XIII.   Make fruit juices and cordials. Evelyn recommends cider and perry, an alcoholic beverage made from the fermented juices of ripened pears

XIV.   Harvest ripe fruits. Fruits thought to be in their prime by Evelyn are: apples, pears, peaches, nectarines, plums, grapes, mulberries, figs, filberts (a type of hazelnut) and yes – melons!

XV.   'Now (and not till now, if you expect success)' warns Evelyn, 'is the just season for the budding of the orange tree.' Well, nothing much has changed there – a vigilant gardener is ever grateful for such providential signs that all will be well in the ensuing growing year and the emergent buds of any perennial are always full of next year's promise

XVI.   Sow hardy seeds. Evelyn favours larkspur, candy-tufts, columbines and 'iron-colour'd fox-gloves, holly-hocks and such plants as endure winter, and the approaching seasons'

XVII.   Finally, Evelyn recommends planting 'anemone roots to have flowers all winter'. Other botanicals Evelyn plants at this time include: musk rose, oleanders, myrtle, starwort, heliotrope, daisies, pansies, nigella, scabius, delphiniums and lupins

Throughout July we are advised to:

V.   Prune shade-producing leaves from fruiting botanicals. Says Evelyn: 'Purge wall fruit of superfluous leaves which hinder from the sun; but do it discreetly'

VI.   Allow seeds for later collection to ripen

VII.   Set wasp traps. Evelyn recommends a glass of beer and honey 'to entice wasps' that would otherwise spoil ripening fruits

VIII.   Take up early autumn bulbs. Evelyn advises: 'Cutting off and trimming the fibres, spread them to air in some dry place'

IX.   Weed gravelled walks and spray with a tobacco and water mixture 'To destroy both worms and weeds, of which it will cure them for some years'

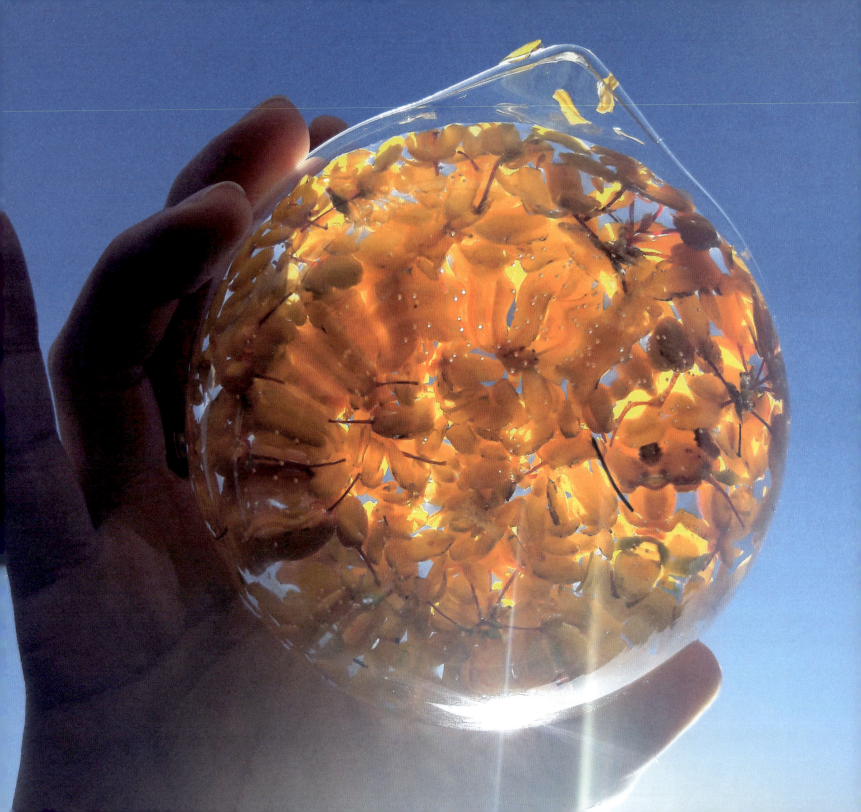

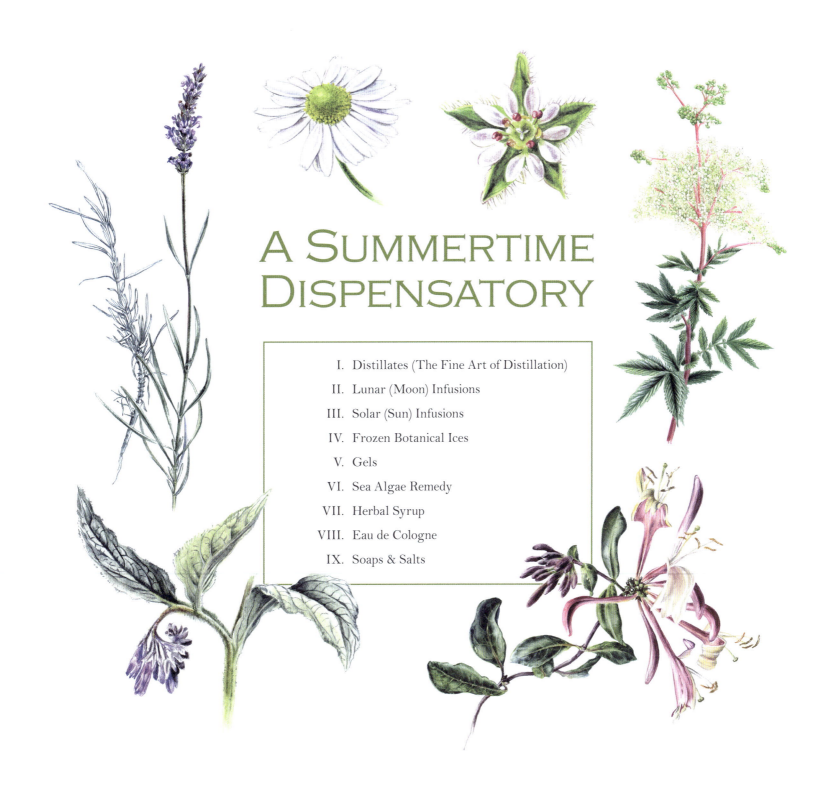

A Summertime Dispensatory

I.
DISTILLATES
(THE FINE ART OF
DISTILLATION)

Before we begin, it should be clearly stated that the most eagerly desired product of all herbology distillation is an aromatic water, rather than an essential oil or alcohol – although we do get a lot of requests for the latter!

The simplest definition of distillation is the method by which the component parts of a liquid (mixture) are separated by selective boiling and condensation. The liquid is then boiled to produce steam and cooled until it condenses back into a liquid. The fine art of distillation originates from and was perfected in Arabia. Traditional alembics (distilling apparatus) were developed in

order to achieve this and over time more sophisticated 'stills' were created and knowledge of distillation dissipated far and wide. During the 17th century, every notable household in England would have had a dedicated 'still room'.

Our herbology distillation classes use beautiful handcrafted copper alembics with wonderful onion bulb shaped lids. These alembics are filled with three quarters of cold water and the selected botanicals (around three times as much water to botanical). The alembics are then heated and we are able to cautiously trace and follow (by feel) the passage of heat as

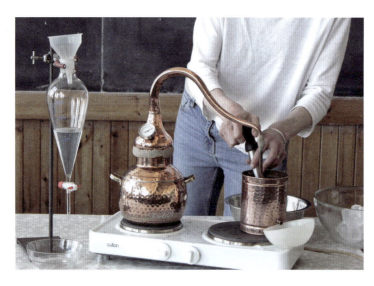
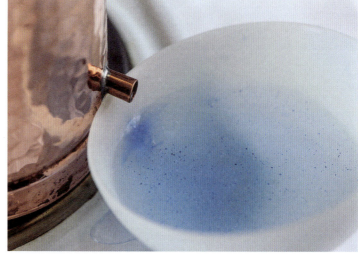

the steam travels through the copper piping. The condensing chambers are then packed with ice and the condensed liquid (now an aromatic water) escapes through an outflow pipe. The aromatic water is captured in a collection bowl or jug and then poured into a separating funnel to be syphoned off from the small amount of essential oil that is tangentially produced.

Although we absolutely love to work with the alembics, some highly successful distillates may be achieved using little more than the most rudimentary of homemade stills cunningly cobbled together from assorted pots and pans – we call this our 'Heath Robinson affair'!

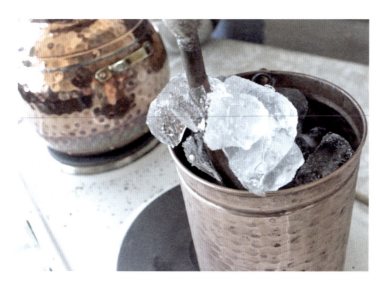

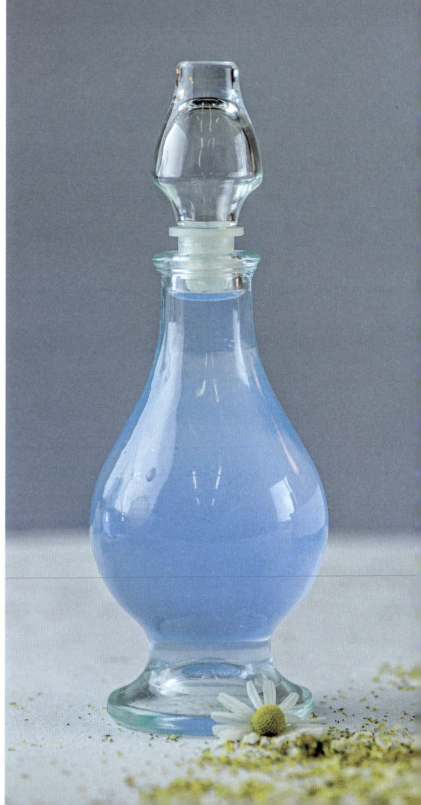

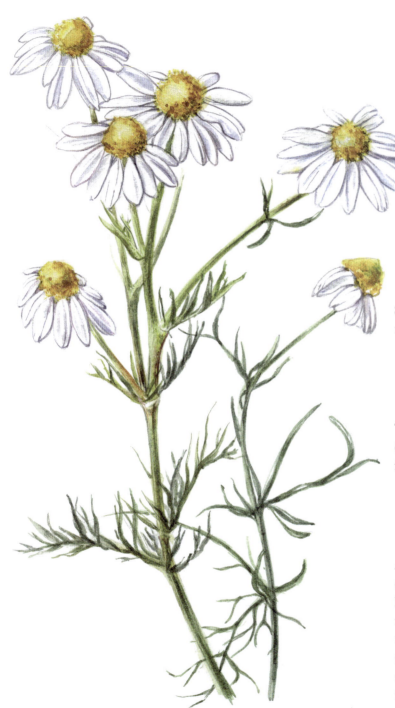

Herbs to Try

Some of our favourite botanicals from the physic garden are reserved for our distillation classes…

Chamomile Flowers

The azulene blue-diffused distillate of wild German chamomile (*Matricaria chamomilla*) is a truly magical thing to create and full of soothing, calming, anti-inflammatory properties.

Lemon Peel

A zingy delight for the senses, the scent of lemon peel (*Citrus limon*) is almost reminiscent of lemon sherbets and its light, invigoratingly uplifting fragrance gives it potential in a refreshing 'perfume spritz' for the summer. Just one little note to be aware of here though: any citrus fruit distillates (just like their essential oils) carry the potential to induce photosensitivity so avoid topical use followed by UV exposure, as this will increase the risk of sunburn.

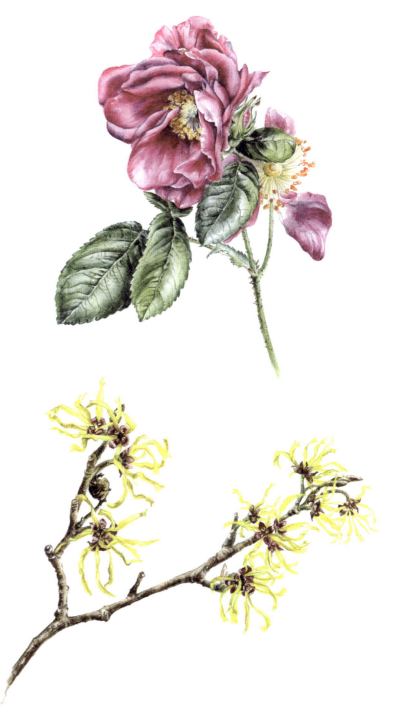

POPLAR BUDS

The sticky, resinous secretions from the buds of the poplar tree (*Populus androscoggin*) scent the western slopes of the Garden with their beguiling balsam-like odour for several intoxicating weeks every year, during which time we eagerly gather those that have fallen around the foot of this magnificent tree.

ROSE PETALS

Perfumed rose petals are the perfect botanicals to choose for your first distillation – use fresh petals and allow the beautiful fragrance captured in the distillate several days to truly 'form' and come together. Don't be put off if your rose distillate resembles boiled cabbage water at first as this will dissipate relatively quickly and transform into something far more wonderful given time!

WITCH HAZEL

A homemade witch hazel (*Hamamelis mollis*) water distillate would be a fun thing to produce. Experiment with the flowers rather than the twiggy parts used in pharmaceutical formulations that are typically distilled in alcohol.

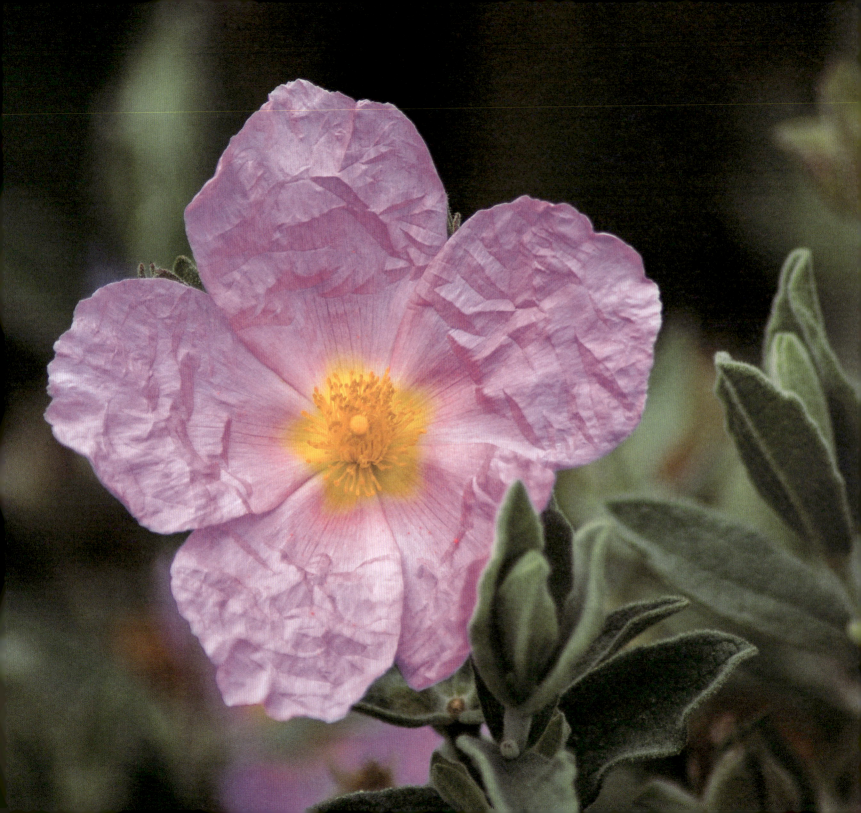

ABOUT AROMATIC WATERS

Aromatic waters are the condensed aqueous product of water or steam distillation. They carry the water-soluble volatile components of the botanical in solution as well as tiny droplets of non-water-soluble essential oils in suspension.

Herbologists distil intentionally to achieve these highly desirable aromatic waters rather than essential oils. For this purpose, we need use only small amounts of our chosen botanicals in 1–3 litre alembics, distilled at low temperatures, with a recognised cut-off point at which we will stop the distillation process so that some remnant volatiles are still left behind in the alembic. This ensures a potent and high-quality aromatic water but a low essential oil yield – exactly what we are after.

With similar properties to essential oils, aromatic waters are believed to hold the very essence (or spirit) of everything that may be found within the botanicals while they are alive but most significantly, they are far less concentrated and therefore potentially far less toxic, with only 0.01–0.1% of dissolved hydrophobic (non-water-soluble) volatile compounds.

HOW TO USE AROMATIC WATERS

Aromatic waters are perhaps at their most delightful when enjoyed as simple odoriferous mists, spritzed lightly into the atmosphere (or upon the face) from a simple pump atomiser. They may be poured into cool summer baths or worked into cosmetic formulations (where they could replace the water element e.g. in lotions, creams, gels or toners). They may even be used diluted as tonics or frozen into ices.

Remember not to heat your aromatic waters, as they are exceptionally delicate (volatile) little creatures and will quite literally vaporise themselves, becoming that tantalisingly elusive 'angel's share' that is so familiar to distillers but is sadly indicative of them being lost to the ether forever.

The following recipe has been adapted with kind permission from Nicola Todd-Macnaughton. You do not need to prepare your own distillate to make this cream – perfectly beautiful rose waters are readily available from most local grocery stores, herbal dispensaries and pharmacies.

This delightfully gentle, cooling and delicately fragranced cream is ideal for soothing the cutaneous tissues during summer.

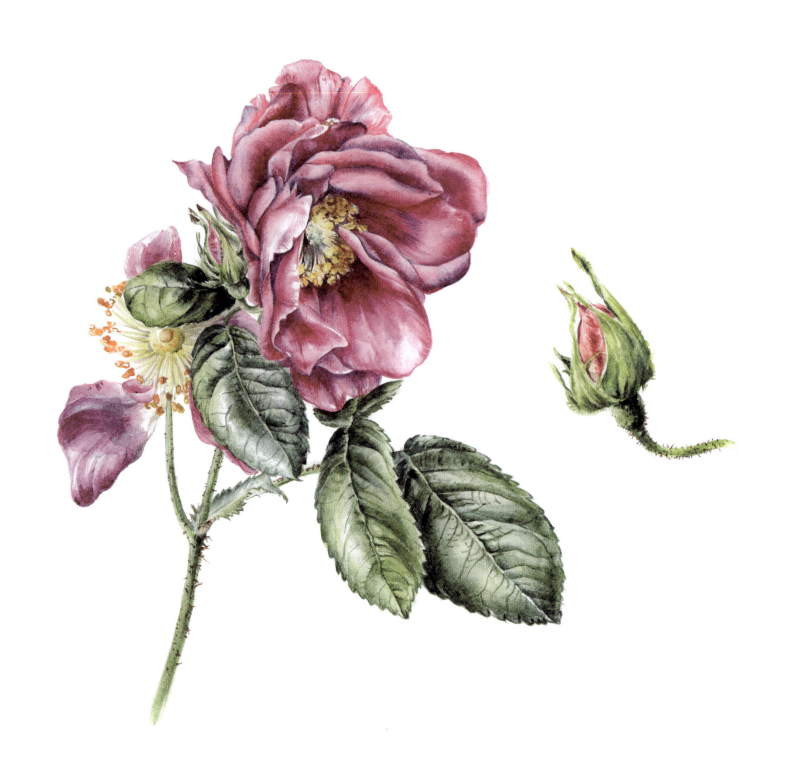

ROSE WATER CREAM RECIPE

INGREDIENTS

30ml organic sweet almond oil

20ml rose petal-infused almond oil

7g unrefined cocoa or shea butter

4g beeswax (or vegan substitute)

40ml rose water distillate
(rose-infused mineral water will suffice)

6g emulsifying wax

Optional: 3–7 drops frankincense essential oil

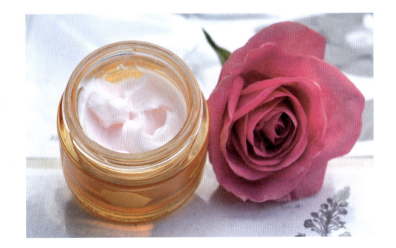

HOW TO MAKE

- Measure out the oils, beeswax and butter and melt together in a bain-marie

- Gently warm the rose water distillate in a separate lidded bain-marie to capture any volatiles that might escape

- Add the emulsifying wax to the rose water and allow to melt

- Remove the oleo-wax mixture from the heat

- Slowly add the rose water and emulsifying wax solution to the oleo-wax solution

- Whip rapidly until cool and the mixture is a soft creamy consistency

- Add a few drops of frankincense essential oil, if using, and stir thoroughly

- Spoon into a 100ml jar

- Lid and label

HOW TO USE

Apply locally as needed to soothe, calm and refresh the cutaneous tissues.

STORAGE

Store this cream in the fridge and use within three weeks or freeze the mixture in ice cube trays to store indefinitely and defrost a cube as required.

Author's note: *If you would like to learn more about how to distil your own botanicals at home, the fascinating chemistry involved and How to Make beautiful 'distilled' products from a range of exquisite aromatic waters, you can study alembic distillation as part of the herbology programme at Royal Botanic Garden Edinburgh. To find out more, please visit our website: rbge.org.uk/learn/short-courses*

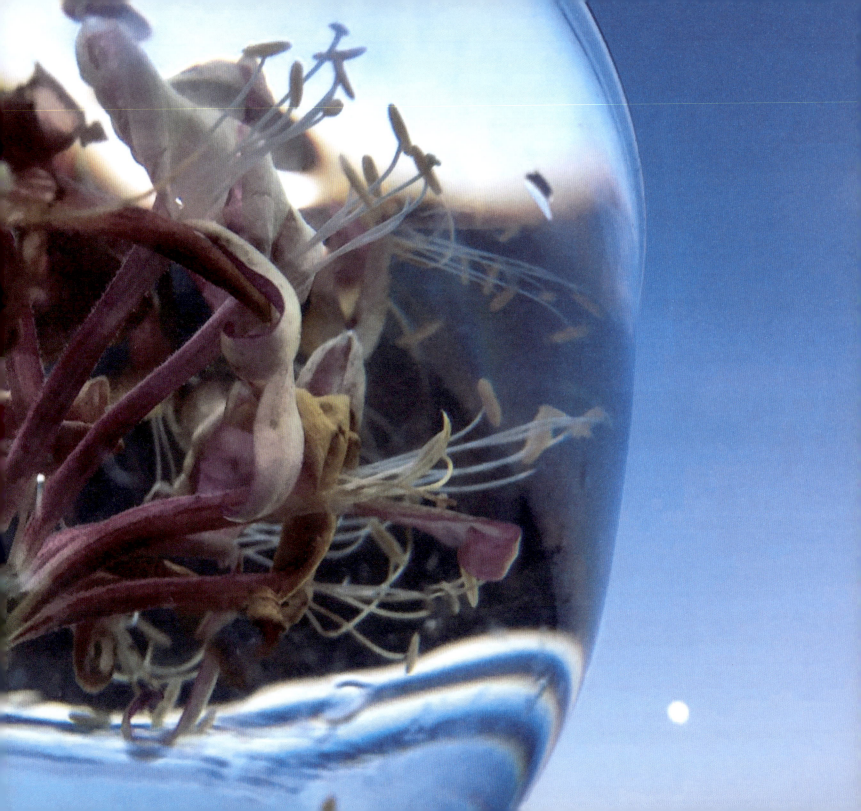

II.

LUNAR (MOON) INFUSIONS

There is nothing that compares (as far as herbology goes) to the ethereal magic of working by the light of the moon, whether that be out in the physic garden or when engaged in our more nocturnal remedy making. So, when our pharmaceutical pursuits naturally turned towards formulations being prepared under the influence of the moon, it was not entirely unexpected.

Our first exhilarating experience of preparing a moon water infusion, conducted after hours in the silent and moonlit grounds of the Garden, took place one unforgettable night. Memories of carrying small glass bowls full of gleaming water topped with goat willow catkins across the silent and deserted moonlit lawns and paths, still thrill those who recall them.

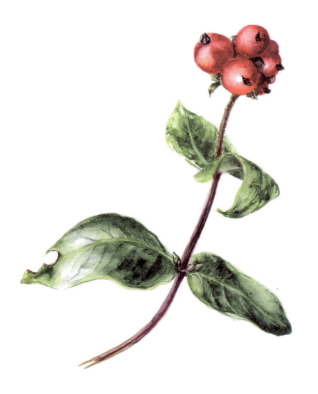

ABOUT
LUNAR INFUSIONS

Lunar infusions are botanical waters imbrued by the light of the moon. They are etheric medicine and belong essentially within the realms of our more esoteric, resonant and spirit-based healing. Intended to nurture the soul rather than the purely physical body, they work on higher, more vibrational frequencies than the other remedies that we use.

It should be noted here that such formulations are rarely approved of by those who require an irrefutably robust, pharmacological evidence-based rationale to account for the curative powers of just about everything, but the enchantment of 'old magick' practices that full moon infusions evoke is beyond refute – at least by those who have experienced it. There is arguably nothing that could afford a truer sense of connection to heaven and earth than this.

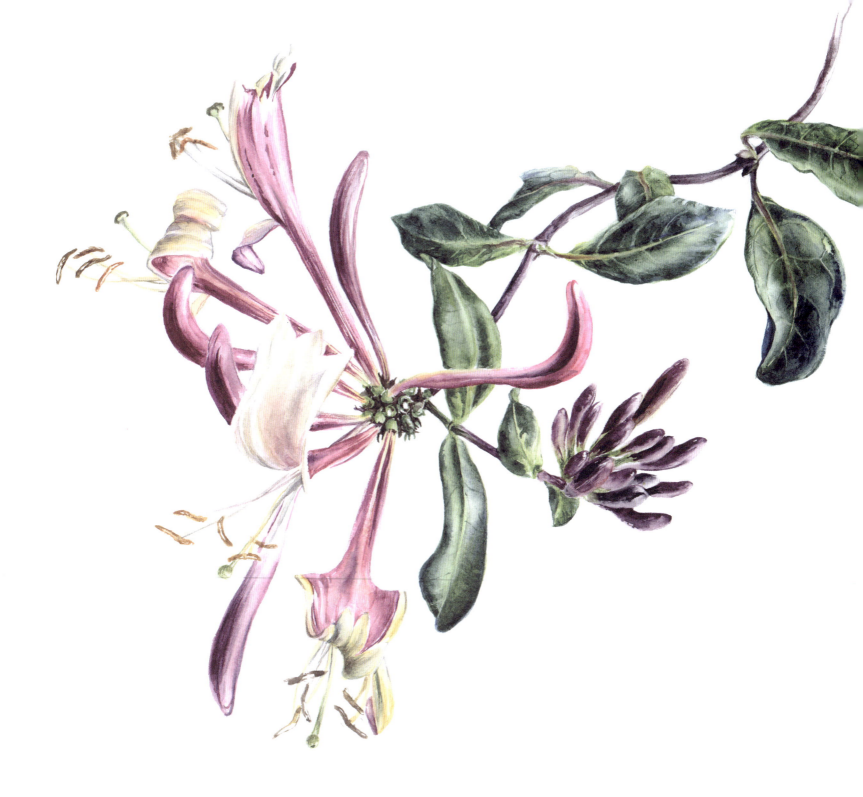

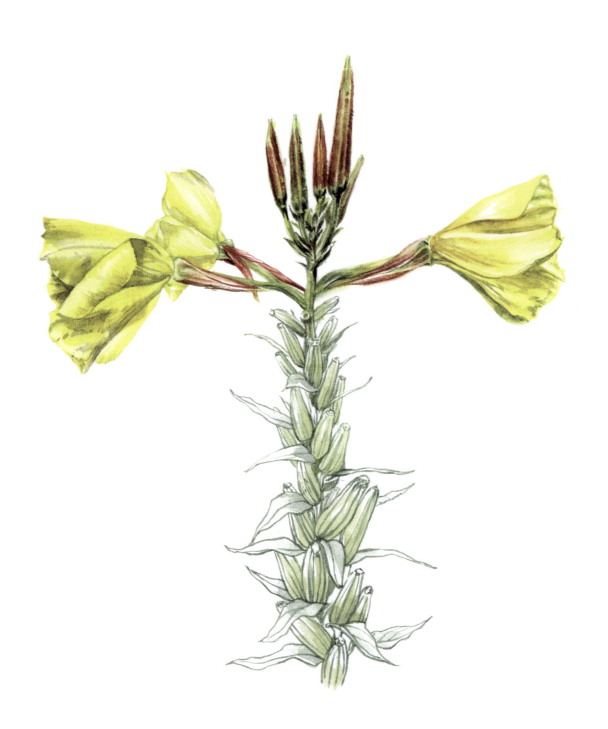

LUNAR INFUSION RECIPE

INGREDIENTS

Cold water, sufficient to fill a small glass bowl – natural spring water is generally preferred but not essential

Botanical flowers (ideally night bloomers, examples listed opposite) to cover the surface area of your bowl

And not forgetting the quintessential element, a full moon! (Ideally a harvest full moon as it's closest to the September equinox)

HERBS TO TRY

- HONEYSUCKLE (*Lonicera periclymenum*) flowers (the berries are toxic)
- NIGHT-SCENTED JASMINE (*Cestrum nocturnum*) flowers
- WHITE-SCENTED ROSE (*Rosa alba*) petals
- EVENING PRIMROSE (*Oenothera biennis*) flowers
- MUGWORT (*Artemisia vulgaris*) aerial parts

Author's note: *Many other botanicals may be used for full moon infusions (both flowers and aerial parts) but as always make sure that whatever you choose is not toxic.*

HOW TO MAKE

- Wait until the full moon rises

- As soon as your garden (or where you wish to conduct your lunar infusion) is bathed in light, fill a clear glass bowl with cold water

- Carefully, and silently, gather the flowers needed to completely cover the surface area of the water

- Be fully aware of your intentions at this moment and breathe in the moonlit night air deeply and slowly, relinquishing any tensions from your heart with every exhalation

- Place the bowl so it stands in full moonlight, unbroken by any shadows

- Leave until dawn the following morning, retrieving your bowl just before sunrise

- Once indoors, strain out the flowers and bottle the moon-infused waters

HOW TO USE

Moon waters may be used in creams, lotions and toners. If sufficient is produced, they ensure an invigorating bathe or body rinse, especially if chilled! They are also perfect for making frozen botanical ices (p. 113). Alternatively, simply imbibe to refresh mind, body and spirit. Moon waters or essences may be created (and preserved) by adding 50% alcohol (e.g. vodka) and pouring the solution into dark glass pipette-stoppered bottles in drop measures to enhance the vibrational properties of any other liquid herbal formulations, or sublingually or diluted in a little spring water.

STORAGE

Refrigerate as soon as it is ready and use within 24 hours, or freeze for later use in herbal remedy making.

Author's note: *Lunary distilling (a corruption of 'lunarie distilling') refers to the moonwort botanical* (Lunaria or Honesty), *with its moon-like seed cases, and comes from a 17th century pastoral poem, 'Nymphidia: The Court of the Fairy' (1627), by Michael Drayton.*

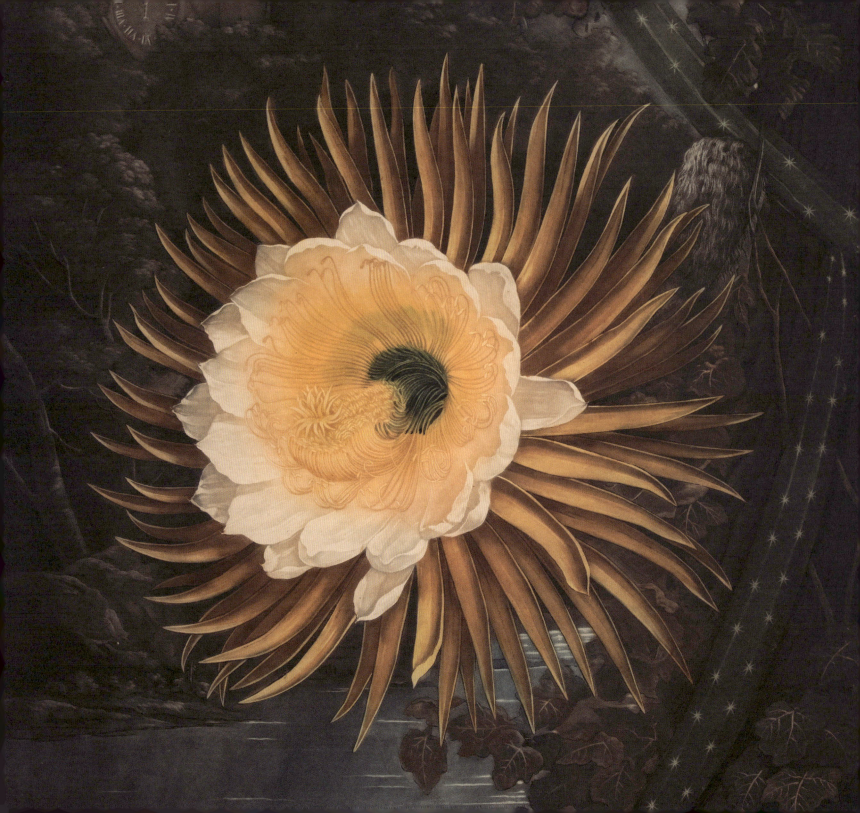

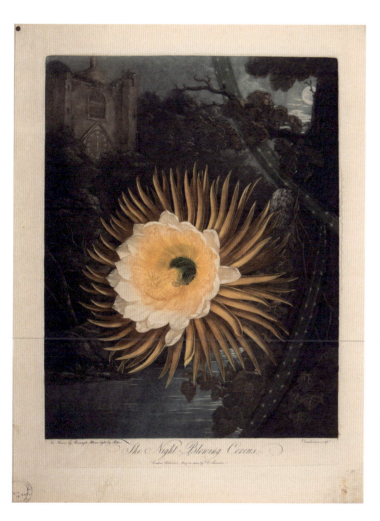

NIGHT-BLOOMING FLOWERS

One glasshouse botanical at the Garden, which has long captured the imagination as a potential and highly desirable botanical for a little 'lunary distilling' of this sort, is the night-blooming cereus (cactus). There are several night-flowering cacti in the glasshouse collection, and it is by all accounts a wonderful sight when they put on their 'flowers by night show' but it's probably only Marley (the resident Garden cat) who gets to see it!

Some, such as *Selenicereus grandiflorus*, bloom only once a year and for one night only, when they will hopefully be pollinated by bats. Imagine if it were possible to gather such a flower on a full moon night and infuse it in a crystal glass of moonlit waters – what a truly magical experience that would be!

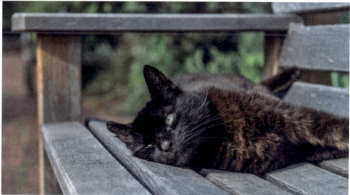

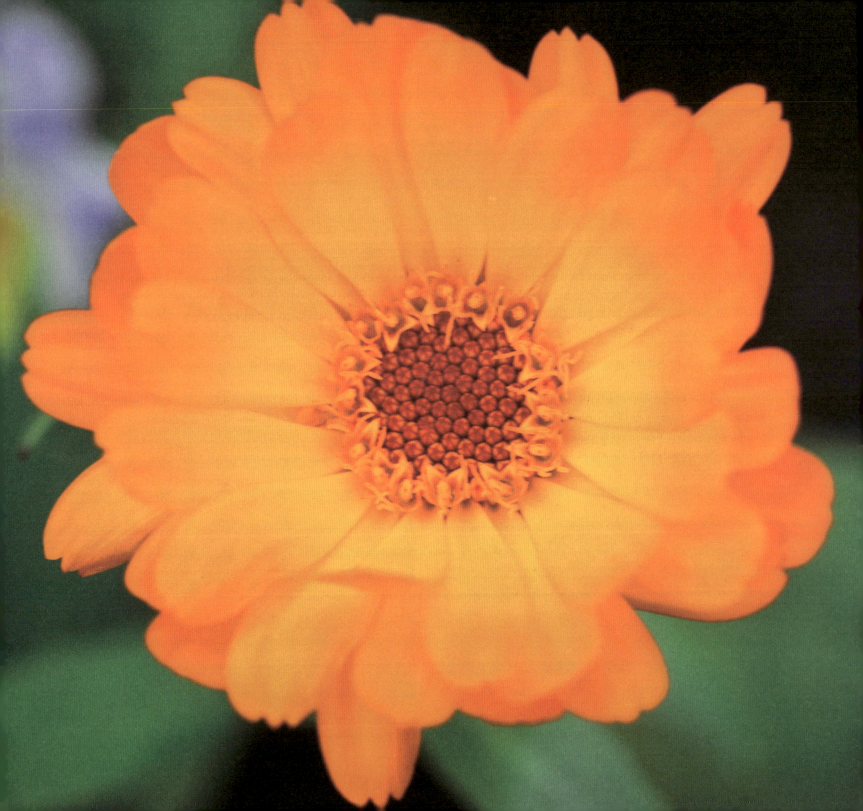

III.
SOLAR (SUN) INFUSIONS

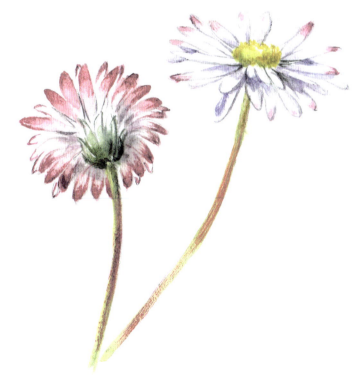

Learning how to infuse flowers in sunlight began as an exploration of the flower essences and in particular the work of Dr Edward Bach. Their preparation is almost identical to that of lunar infusions but with one notable exception – these are botanical waters infused by the light of the sun.

They are intended to work on the same etheric level as botanical moon waters, freeing an individual of the psychological impediments that may be 'holding them back' from their true selves.

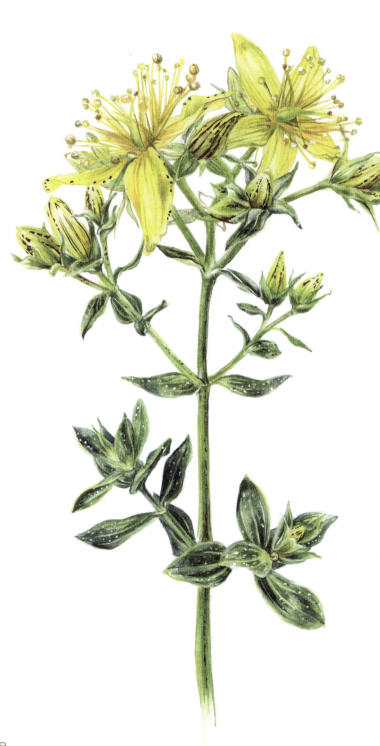

SOLAR INFUSION
RECIPE

INGREDIENTS

Cold water, sufficient to fill a small glass bowl –
natural spring water is generally preferred
but not essential

Botanical flowers to cover
the surface area of your bowl

Sun – although cloudless blue heavens are definitely
advocated for achieving the ideal solar infusion,
our Edinburgh herbologists have discovered a perfectly
acceptable alternative now fondly referred to as a
'cloud infusion'

HERBS TO TRY

- ST JOHN'S WORT (*Hypericum perforatum*)
- CALIFORNIAN POPPIES (*Eschscholzia californica*)
- CORNFLOWERS (*Centaurea cyanus*)
- DAISIES (*Bellis perennis*)
- GRASS-OF-PARNASSUS (*Parnassia palustris*)

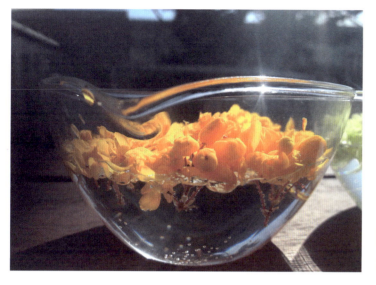

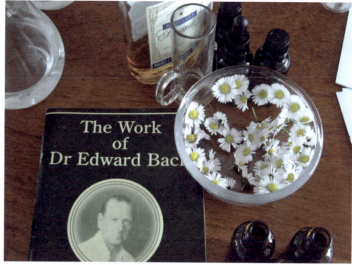

How to Make

- As soon as your garden (or where you wish to conduct your solar infusion) is bathed in light, fill a clear glass bowl with cold water

- Carefully, and silently, gather the flowers needed to completely cover the surface area of the water

- Be fully aware of your intentions at this moment and breathe in deeply and slowly, relinquishing any tensions from your heart with every exhalation

- Place the bowl so it stands in the sun, unbroken by any shadows

- Leave until night falls, retrieving your bowl just before the sun sets

- Once indoors, strain out the flowers and bottle the solar-infused waters

How to Use

Solar waters may be used in cosmetic and/or herbal creams, lotions and toners. If sufficient is produced, they ensure an invigorating bathe or body rinse, especially if chilled! They are also perfect for making frozen botanical ices (p. 113). Alternatively, simply imbibe to refresh mind, body and spirit. On a far more practical level, solar waters or essences may be created (and preserved) by adding 50% alcohol (e.g. vodka) and pouring the solution into dark glass pipette-stoppered bottles. These may be added in drop measures to enhance the vibrational properties of any other liquid herbal formulations, or else enjoyed entirely by themselves taken sublingually or diluted in a little spring water.

Storage

This water should be refrigerated as soon as it is ready, and used within 24 hours, or alternatively it may be stored frozen for later use in herbal remedy making.

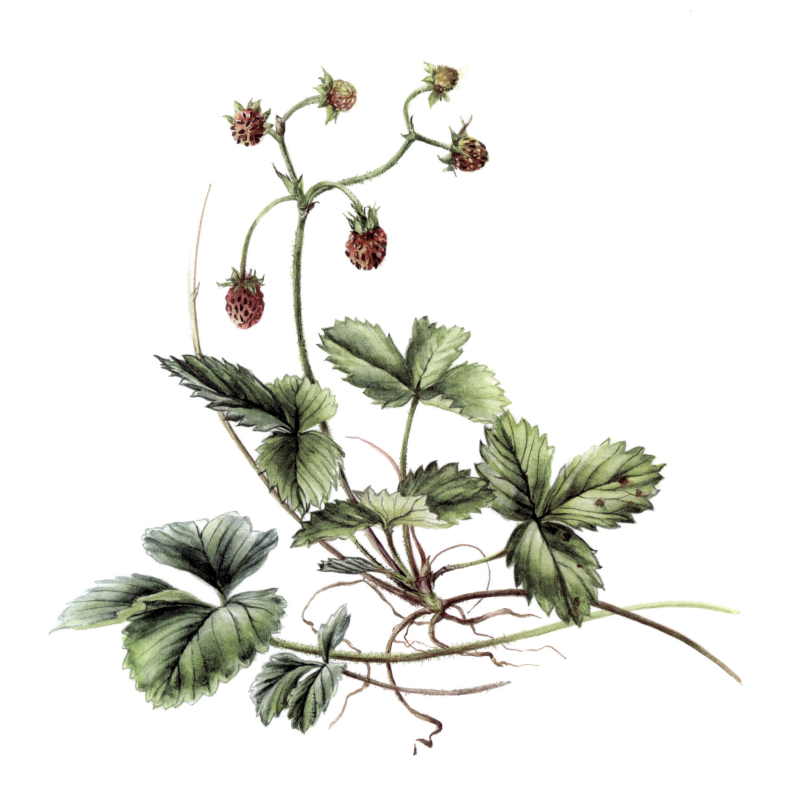

IV.
FROZEN BOTANICAL ICES

An enchanting early summer alternative to our herbal infusion repertoire (of celestial origin or not) are these delightfully refreshing 'ices', which may be made using either just pure water or the aqueous extracts described earlier.

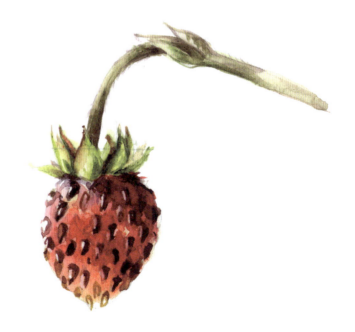

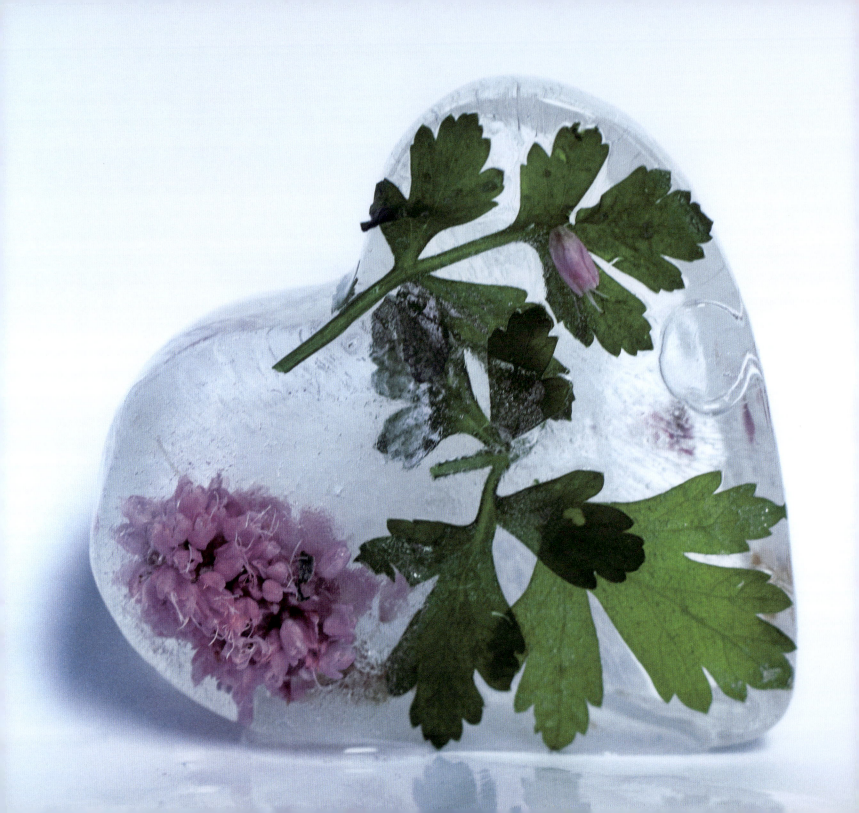

Botanical Ices
Recipe

Ingredients

Your chosen botanicals and extracts (see below)

Fresh cold water

Silicone moulds

Herbs to Try

- HEARTSEASE (*Viola tricolor*) flowers
- PARSLEY (*Petroselinum crispum*) leaf
- BLACK LACE ELDER (*Sambucus nigra*) flowers
- FENNEL (*Foeniculum vulgare*) leaf
- BORAGE (*Borago officinalis*) flowers
- CHAMOMILE (*Matricaria chamomilla*) leaf and flowers
- LOVE-IN-A-MIST (*Nigella damascena*) flowers
- ROSE (*Rosa damascea*) petals
- MARIGOLD (*Calendula officinalis*) flowers
- BLACKCURRANT (*Ribes nigrum*) leaf and berry clusters
- CORNFLOWERS (*Centaurea cyanus*) flowers
- BLACK PEPPERMINT (*Mentha piperita*) leaf
- HIBISCUS (*Hibiscus* sp.) flowers
- PASSIONFLOWER (*Passiflora incarnata*) aerial parts
- HOPS (*Humulus lupulus*) leaf and tendrils
- SEA BUCKTHORN (*Hippophae rhamnoides*) leaf and berries
- WILD STRAWBERRY (*Fragaria vesca*) leaf, runners, flowers, fruit

How to Make

- Gather the desired botanicals
- Put a selection in cold water and store in the fridge for later use
- Using 3 tsp of fresh herb per 1 cup water, infuse the remaining botanicals for 5–10 minutes
- Strain out the botanicals
- Allow to cool
- Remove the botanicals from the fridge
- Place decorative pieces of the botanicals in the bottom of silicone moulds
- Pour enough to half fill the moulds and freeze
- Once frozen, top up the moulds with the remaining infusion
- Freeze again to capture all the botanicals entirely in ice

How to Take

These frozen extracts are quite beautiful when added to another cold-water herbal infusion, syrup cordial or traditional British Pimm's.

Storage

Store in an icebox until required.

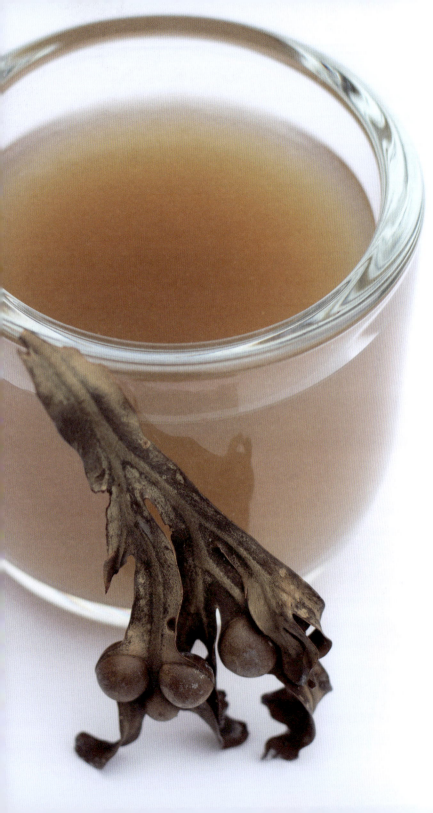

V.
GELS

There is nothing quite so soothing in the heat of summer as the application of a cooling (chilled from the fridge) botanical-based gel. There are several different types of gel, with colloidal and/or hydrogels generally being the ones most frequently encountered and used therapeutically. Gels are fascinating translucent mediums that exist somewhere between a liquid and a solid. Generally comprised mostly of liquid, they have a viscosity that enables them to behave like loosely formed solids. They are exceptionally healing in a very gentle way and may be used with care on wounds, burns and – dependent upon their nature – some may even be taken orally.

Here is a very simple recipe for a classic sea algae gel that we prepare every year. It can be used alone as an emollient topical vulnerary but its inherently medicinal nature may be greatly enhanced by various adjuncts, which are noted overleaf. For our herbologists, the gel extraction is only the first step in a formulation that may be further developed into an exquisite cream.

The sea algae used to make this gel is carrageen (*Chondrus crispus*), one of our shore's most beautiful red seaweeds.

Author's note: *An easy to source alternative to the carrageen would be agar agar – another of the gelatinous sea algae, available in most good grocery and health food stores. Just follow the instructions on the packet to make a very similar base gel.*

CARRAGEEN GEL EXTRACT RECIPE

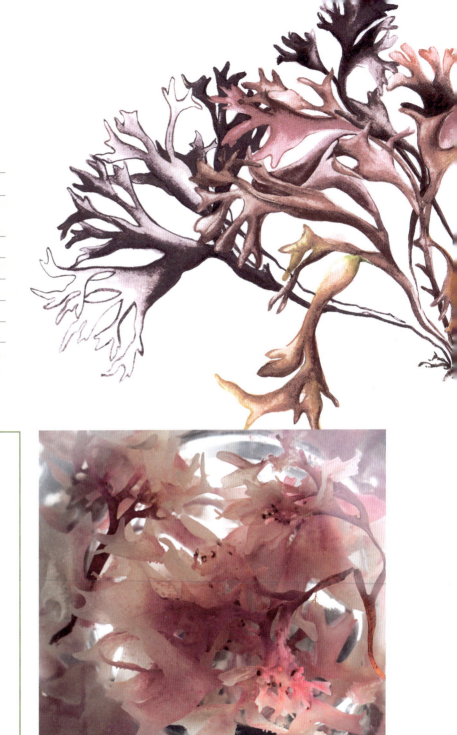

INGREDIENTS

1 part carrageen to 40 parts cold water

OPTIONAL INGREDIENTS

Botanical infusions, decoctions or vulnerary green juices

Aromatic waters

Lunar or solar infusions

Alcoholic herbal extracts (e.g. witch hazel)

A few drops of essential oil

Around 5ml of any of the above (with the exception of the essential oil) may be added to 30ml gel (depending on the consistency required), or 3–5 drops essential oil

HOW TO MAKE

- Place the carrageen and water in a heavy-bottomed pot
- Slowly heat the water until it bubbles gently around the carrageen – a gel will readily be released
- After 20 minutes, strain out the rubbery remnants of carrageen

HOW TO USE

While the application of just pure and unadulterated gels will impart a comforting and therapeutic lubrication to underlying tissues, the addition of a few other simple ingredients will make it doubly efficacious and medicinal.

STORAGE

Gels (being aqueous extracts) are best stored frozen.

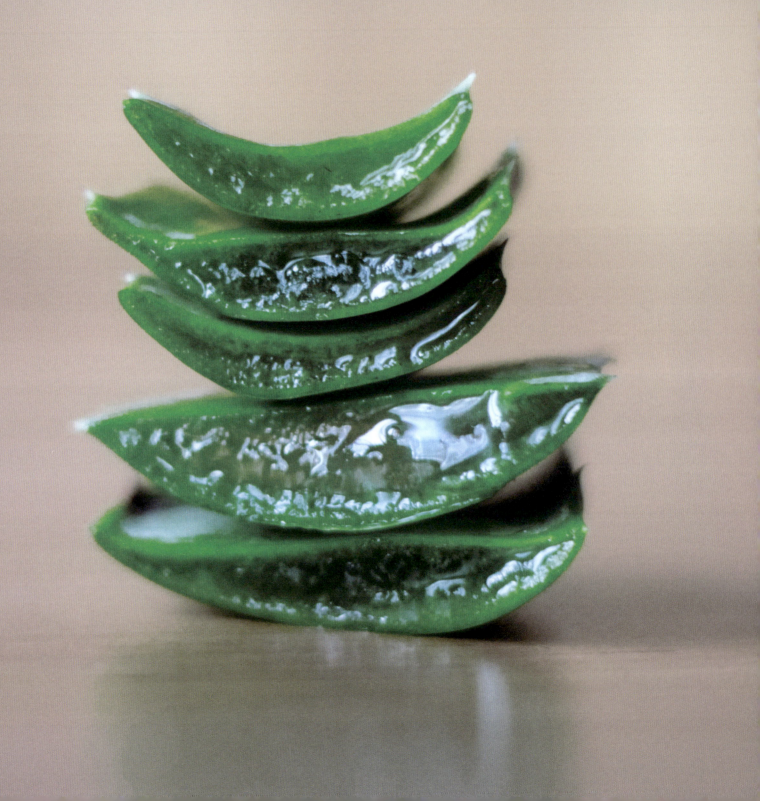

ALOE GEL CREAM

Another of the lightest and most readily absorbed formulations for the summer is this cooling aloe vera gel-based cream, which may be used to calm hot, inflamed or sunburnt cutaneous tissues. The recipe below is infinitely adaptable, dependent upon which of the liquid extracts (waters) and oils are incorporated into the gel base.

ALOE GEL CREAM RECIPE

INGREDIENTS

30g aloe vera gel
(or other gel of your choice)

5ml liquid herbal extract
(e.g. lavender or chamomile water)

5ml infused herbal oil
(e.g. lavender, chamomile, marigold, chickweed, hypericum)

3 drops lavender (or other soothing) essential oil

HERBAL EXTRACTS/ WATERS TO TRY

- WITCH HAZEL, for a cooling and antiseptic effect
- ROSE, to soothe
- LAVENDER, to calm
- CHAMOMILE, for anti-inflammatory properties
- PEPPERMINT, to cool and refresh

HOW TO MAKE

- Spoon the correct measure of aloe vera gel into a 50ml glass jar
- Add the other ingredients
- Mix thoroughly together
- Lid and label

HOW TO USE

Apply as needed to help heal simple wounds, cuts and grazes.

STORAGE

Refrigerate and use within three months.

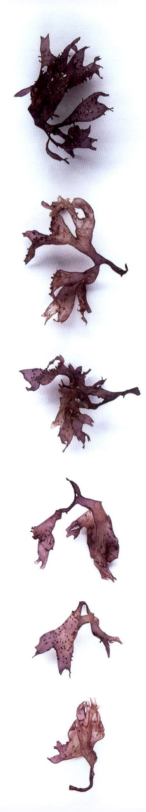

VI.

SEA ALGAE REMEDY

Of all the oceanic delights that will nourish our bodies both nutritionally and therapeutically, there's probably nothing quite so comforting as a homemade 'cream of the ocean' smoothed lightly over the cutaneous tissues. One of the most gently nurturing and soothing of the sea algae creams around, this recipe is brought to you by kind permission of Monica Wilde. This cream formulation has an unusual goat's milk twist, a homage to the traditional blancmange-like puddings that carrageen was once widely used for in the Highlands and Islands.

Author's note: *If you would like to learn more about seaweeds, how to identify and safely forage for seaweed remedies and recipes, book a place on Seaweedopedia, which runs every year as part of the herbology programme at Royal Botanic Garden Edinburgh. To find out more, please visit our website: rbge.org.uk/learn/short-courses*

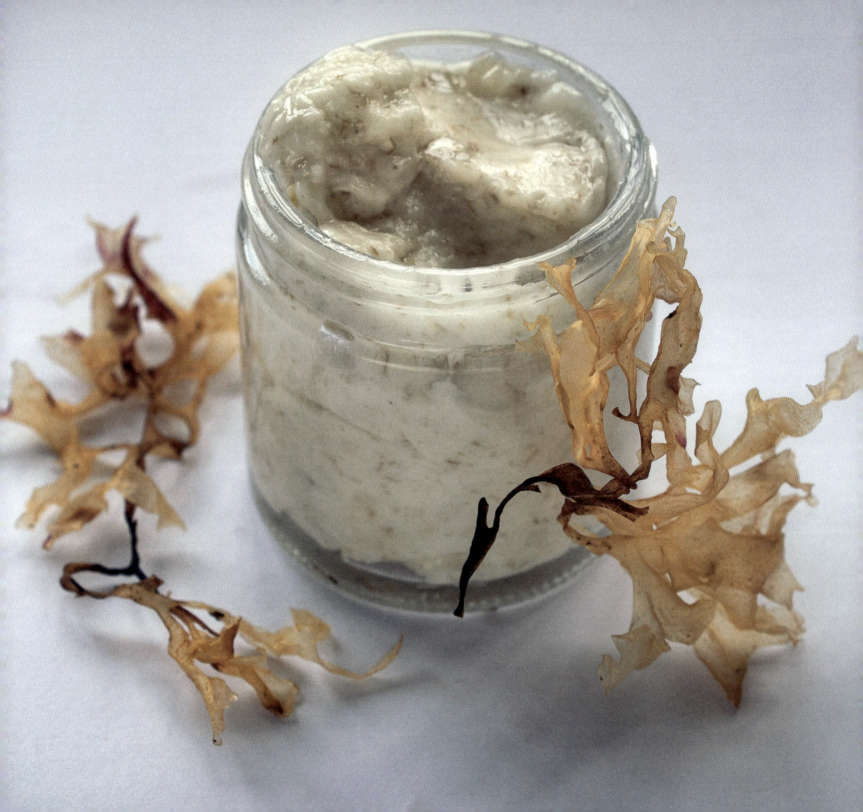

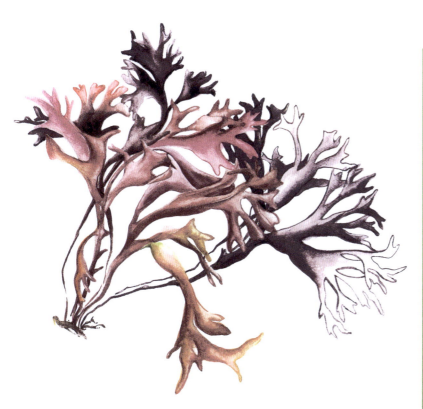

CARRAGEEN & GOAT'S MILK CREAM RECIPE

INGREDIENTS

1.2l (2 pints) water

A good handful of carrageen sea algae

200ml goat's milk (dried vulnerary botanicals may be infused within this, if desired)

100ml oil infused with the vulnerary herb of your choice

Ethylhexylglycerin (always add 1% of total amount of resultant liquid solution)

HOW TO MAKE

- Soak the carrageen in half the water until rubbery and 'plumptious'
- Gently warm the milk in a small pan – add any dry botanicals to create a light infusion – put to one side
- Strain the carrageen and add to a fresh 600ml measure of water in a separate pan
- Bring to the boil and simmer for around 20 minutes, until the water becomes 'gloopy'. Rewarm the milk a little if it has gone cold – the two should be around the same temperature (precision not necessary)
- Strain the carrageen through a strainer or ideally squeeze through a jelly bag (rubber gloves may be required as it can be too hot to handle!)
- Whisk the resulting carrageen gel into the milk infusion
- Drizzle in the infused oil, whisking rapidly
- Add the preservative (if using) and stir thoroughly
- Pour into pots
- Leave to cool
- Lid and label

HOW TO USE

Carrageen cream is a truly pampering and emollient therapy for any tired, dry or damaged tissues, but it's especially beneficial for the face and hands when a little extra love is required.

STORAGE

Keep refrigerated. If no preservative has been added, pour the mixture into ice cube trays and freeze for later use.

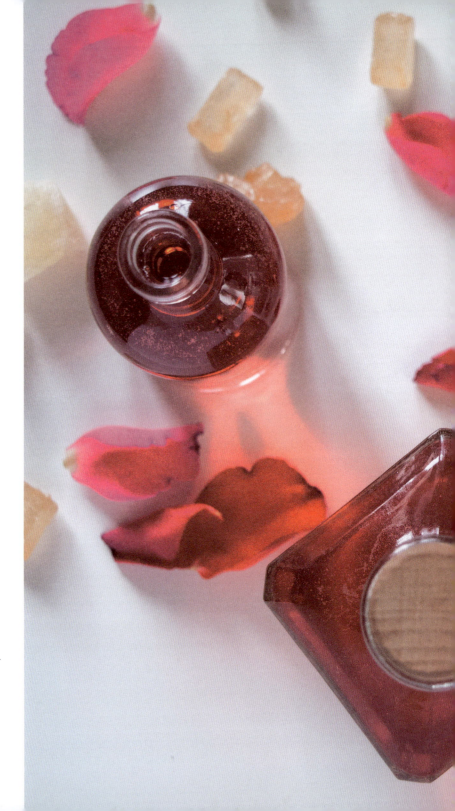

VII.
HERBAL SYRUP

A herbal syrup makes a delicious remedy. Syrups release their potent therapeutic extracts readily into the bloodstream and can help to fortify the immune system and boost the body's energy reserves when depleted.

This sugar or honey-based preparation uses rose petals together with hawthorn flowers and/or fruits as key ingredients – a wonderfully synergistic and aromatic combination. Rose is one of the most delightful botanicals of our pharmacopoeia, believed 'to raise the spirits and cheer the heart' while imparting cooling anti-inflammatory, mildly anaesthetic, sedative, antiviral and antiseptic properties. It is the perfect complement to hawthorn – a true heart tonic, antioxidant and restorative, with a local traditional use to soothe sore throats. Hawthorn is associated with the Celtic fire festival of Beltane, with love and betrothal, while rose is considered an aphrodisiac.

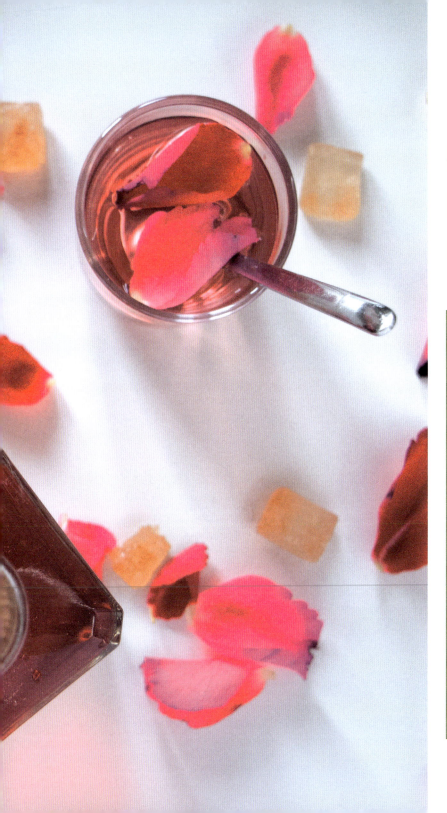

ROSE PETAL SYRUP RECIPE

INGREDIENTS

Hawthorn berry decoction
(all 3 aqueous extracts should equal 500ml of liquid in total)

Hawthorn flower infusion

Rose petal infusion

500g honey or raw cane sugar

HOW TO MAKE

- In a standard syrup recipe use equal parts of sugar to liquid
- An infusion for use in a syrup needs to be steeped for at least 10 minutes, while a decoction may be simmered for around 20 minutes to an hour. Hawthorn berries should be crushed gently in a pestle and mortar before being decocted and simmered for 20 minutes
- Pour the herbal infusions and decoction into a pan
- Add the sugar or honey and warm gently until dissolved
- Remove from the heat and allow to cool
- Pour into sterilised glass bottles using a funnel
- Lid (with a cork) and label

HOW TO TAKE

Take one teaspoon three times daily.

STORAGE

Syrups generally keep for up to six months if refrigerated.

Author's note: *Syrups can ferment and a bottle with a screw top lid may explode – corks are therefore recommended!*

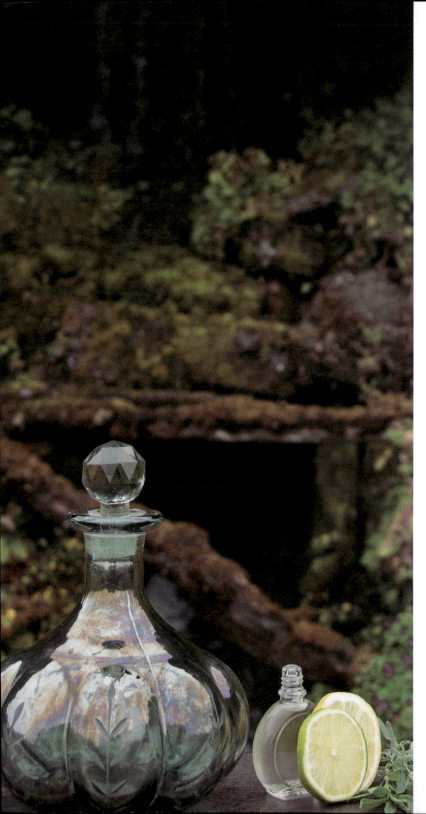

VIII.

EAU DE COLOGNE

We wanted to include something that would be 'pleasantly different' within the pages of this book, so here it is – our eau de cologne.

Eau de cologne, as the name would suggest, originates from Germany, where it was created in 1709 by Italian perfumier Johann Maria Farina. Its subtle, refreshingly light citrus fragrance was one of the earliest perfumes of its kind and is still very much enjoyed in more contemporary perfumery interpretations, especially during the summer when its cooling (refrigerant) effects may be applied to the pulse points for a quick burst of exhilarating fragrance. One of the lovely things about eau de cologne is that it is an ambiguous perfume that may be enjoyed by everyone. Typically comprised of a mixture of zingy citrus oils (try lemon, lime, grapefruit, clementine, tangerine, sweet and bitter orange, bergamot or neroli), together with other oils such as lavender, thyme, rosemary, oregano, jasmine, oleaster, petitgrain – the list is endless.

Here's one especially refreshing formulation for you to try, albeit with a little herbology twist to the ingredients!

Cooling Eau de Cologne Recipe

Ingredients

150ml (half a cup) of vodka

⅛ tsp lemon extract or sweet orange oil

¼ tsp bergamot essential oil

¼ tsp lavender essential oil

⅛ tsp glycerine (or castor oil, cornflour or orris root powder – the latter help with dispersion of the oils in the solution; orris root is a noted fixative used in perfumery)

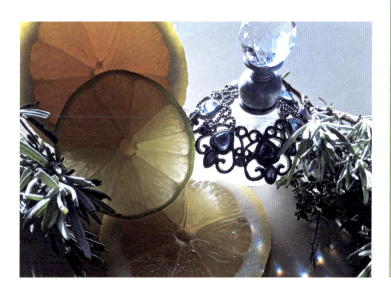

How to Make

- Mix everything together in a glass or ceramic pot/jar
- Cover with a lid
- Allow ingredients to infuse for 1 week in a cool, dark place
- Decant the cologne into a decorative glass bottle or atomiser
- Allow to 'rest' for a further week before using

How to Use

Spritz lightly over the body (apparently the very best way to apply a fragrance) or use your fingers to dab a little onto pulse points.

Storage

This essential oil-infused eau de cologne will retain its fragrance for several years if kept somewhere cool and dark in deep blue or amber glass storage bottles.

Author's note: *This cologne formulation may be easily adapted but it provides a useful guideline for the recommended ratio of essential oil to alcohol. A word of caution: citrus oil is known to cause photosensitivity, please do not use this cologne in the sun.*

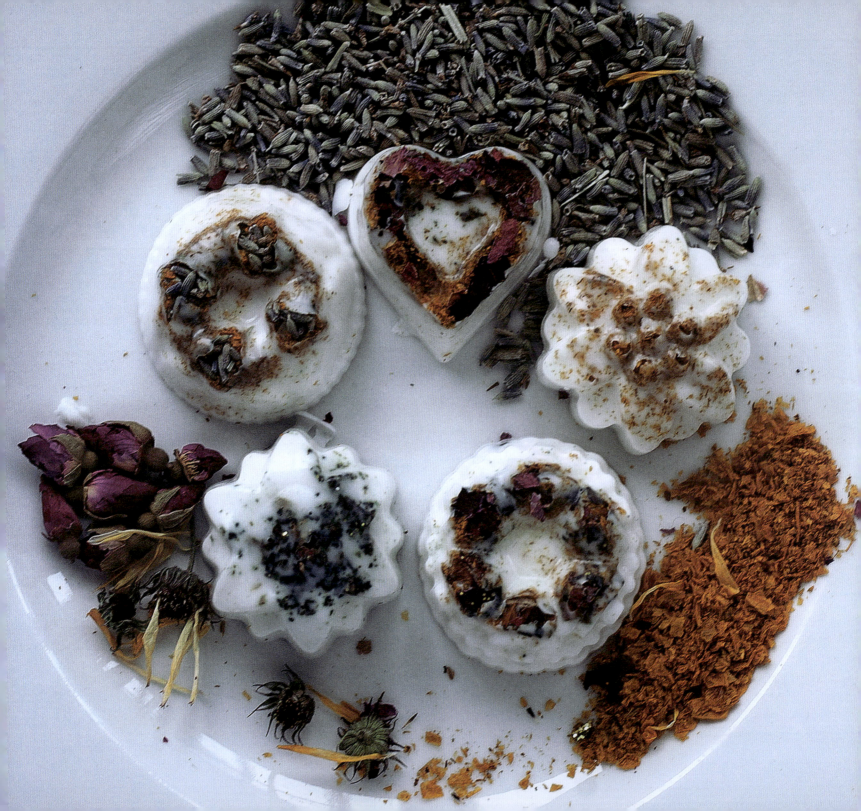

IX.
SOAPS & SALTS

SOAPS
(MELT & POUR)

Our herbology programme has enjoyed many happy (and not entirely uneventful) years of castile soap making under the ever-good-humoured guidance of Caurnie Soaperie. We adapted a very simple 'melt & pour' technique for our Millefleure – Soaps & Salts short course, yielding some of our most easily prepared and decorative cleansing bars, studded as they always are with jewel-like herbaria and botanical fragments.

All that you need are 'melt & pour' soap bases (we use organic crystal clear and goat's milk blocks) which can be sourced from several suppliers – for more information we recommend visiting thesoapkitchen.co.uk.

As with all soap making, you can choose to make a small or big batch depending on your own requirements but an initial order of a 1kg block of 'melt & pour' base provides just sufficient to experiment with – and you can always buy more!

A NOTE ON BOTANICALS IN
SOAPS & SALTS

- Botanical ingredients should always be dried
- You may use flowers, petals and leaves finely powdered and simply stirred through solutions or mixtures
- Use to bejewel your soaps as adornments, sprinkles or pigments (e.g. crushed hibiscus flowers)

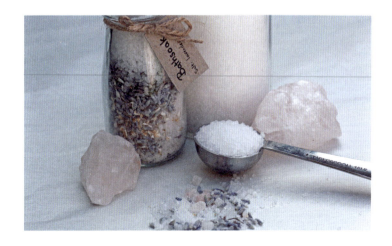

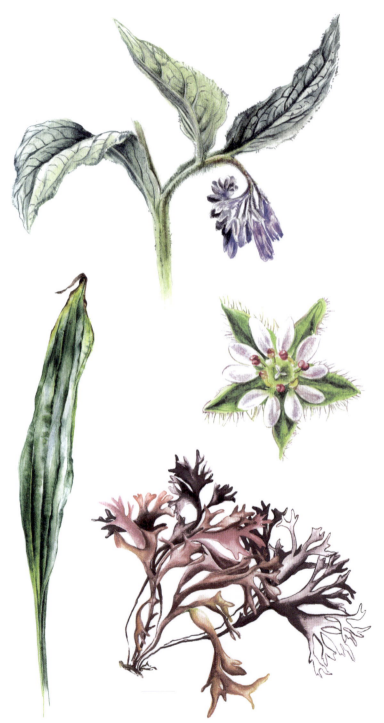

HERBS TO TRY

(Any of the vulnerary herbs (pp. 34–37) are perfectly suited to this purpose)

- ROSE (*Rosa damascena*)
- LAVENDER (*Lavandula angustifolia*)
- CARRAGEEN (*Chondrus crispus*)
- COMFREY (*Symphytum officinale*)
- CHAMOMILE (*Matricaria chamomilla*)
- LADY'S MANTLE (*Alchemilla vulgaris*)
- MARIGOLD (*Calendula officinalis*)
- MARSHMALLOW (*Althaea officinalis*)
- NETTLE (*Urtica dioica*)
- OATS (*Avena sativa*)
- PLANTAIN (*Plantago lanceolata*)
- YARROW (*Achillea millefolium*)
- CHICKWEED (*Stellaria media*)
- DAISY (*Bellis perennis*)
- WITCH HAZEL (*Hamamelis virginiana*)
- ST JOHN'S WORT (*Hypericum perforatum*)
- PEPPERMINT (*Mentha piperita*)

A Note on Essential Oils in Soaps & Salts

- Use essential oils sparingly – just a few drops per soap or handful of salts is usually sufficient

- Essential oils should always complement or enhance the therapeutic effects of other botanicals used in your formulations

A small selection of popular herbology choices
(Each of the following may be used singly or in simple synergistic blends)

- ROSE (*Rosa damascena*)

- LAVENDER (*Lavandula angustifolia*)

- CITRUS (*Citrus* sp.)

- PEPPERMINT (*Mentha* sp.)

- TEA TREE (*Melaleuca alternifolia*)

- THYME (*Thymus* – thyme and lime is a herbology favourite and a truly invigorating combination!)

- PINE (*Pinus*)

- EUCALYPTUS (*Eucalyptus globulus*)

- CHAMOMILE (*Matricaria chamomilla*)

- SANDALWOOD (*Santalum album*)

- FRANKINCENSE (*Olibanum*)

- WINTERGREEN (*Gaultheria procumbens*)

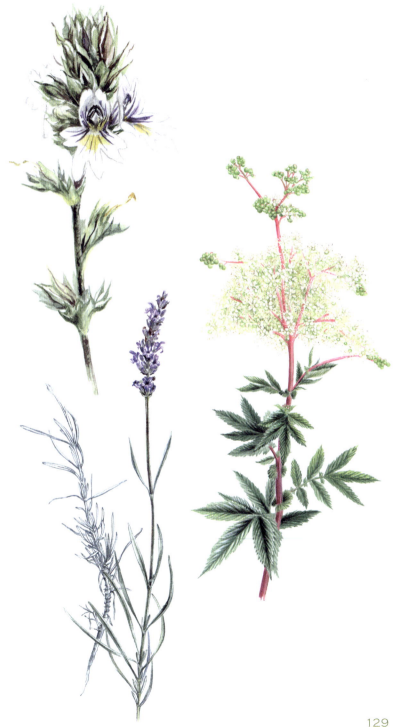

A 'MELT & POUR' SOAP RECIPE

INGREDIENTS

½–1 block 'melt & pour' soap base

1 handful dried herbal flowers and their petals

Optional: a few drops of essential oil fragrances

Optional: a few drops of pigment colour –
less is often more!

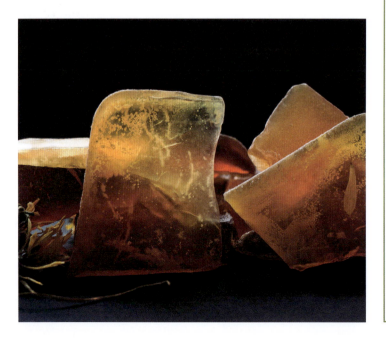

HOW TO MAKE

- Cut the 'melt & pour' soap base into small lumps and place in a bain-marie

- Warm until the lumps melt and liquify

- Remove from the heat

- Add the dried botanicals, fragrances and pigment colours

- Pour into moulds

- Allow to cool and set

HOW TO USE

Use as decorative alternatives to regular soaps.

STORAGE

Remove from moulds and wrap in waxed paper for storage until required.

Author's note: *The dried botanicals, fragrances, pigment colours etc. may be added to the melted soap base either before or after pouring into the moulds.*

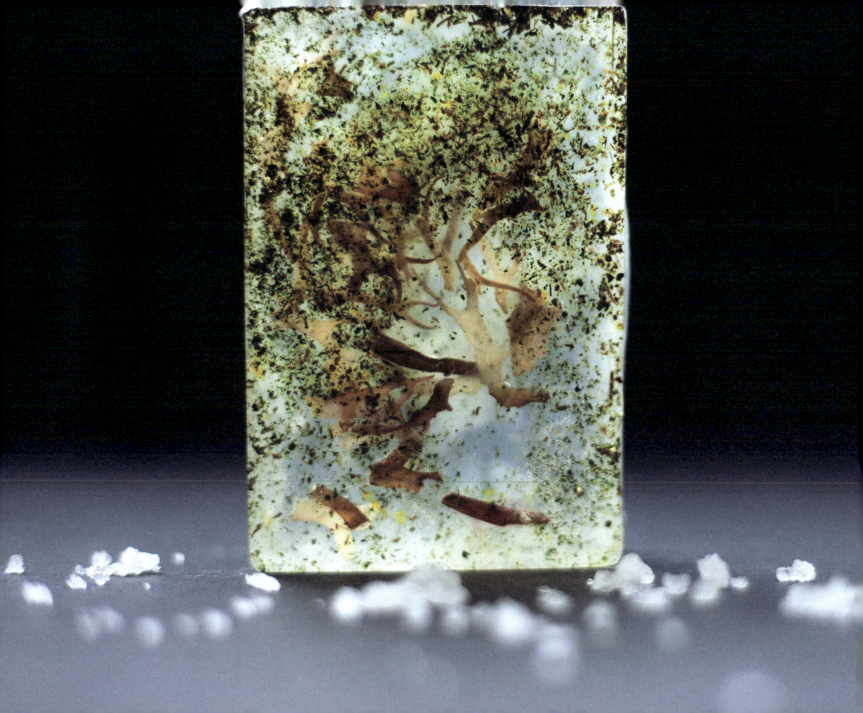

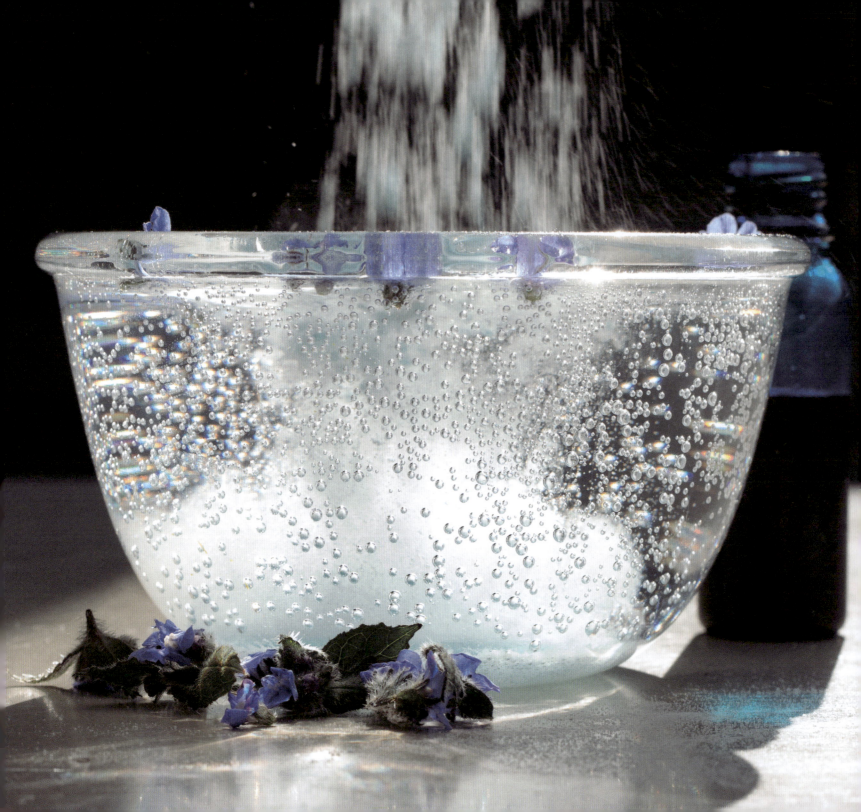

SALTS

Sometimes, in the hot languorous days of high summer, we just need to have a little refreshingly frivolous fun. Adding some bubbles and fizz to an otherwise perfectly acceptable bath salts remedy may seem an indulgent herbology frivolity, but is it really? Not quite! The combined effects of the salts, citric acid and bicarbonate of soda in the following bathing formulation produce some synergistically charged and therapeutically complementary effects.

The slightly salty, alkaline bicarbonate of soda is a naturally cleansing agent, with antiseptic, anti-inflammatory and gently exfoliant properties – simply adding a couple of cups to a bath, allowing it to dissolve slowly and soaking in its soothing solution for half an hour or so may relieve many minor cutaneous tissue irritations.

The citric acid powder (completely safe to use in this sort of dilution) is the essential element required to achieve the fizzy effervescent effects that we are after. Sea salts, with or without powdered seaweeds, yield deeply therapeutic effects during a deep bathing soak and are full of detoxifying and re-mineralising potential.

So, here follows the most light-hearted of our remedy selection, for a little fun (fizzing!) bath time delight.

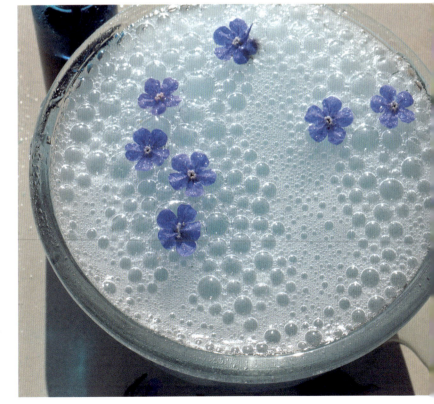

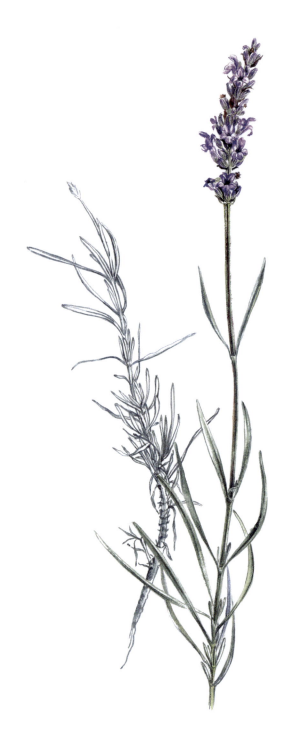

FIZZING SUMMER BATH SALTS RECIPE

INGREDIENTS

1 cup sea salt crystals

½ cup bicarbonate of soda

¼ cup citric acid powder

5–8 drops essential oil (e.g. rose or lavender)

3–5 drops natural liquid pigment

Dried botanicals – these are optional but plug hole strainers will be required if used!

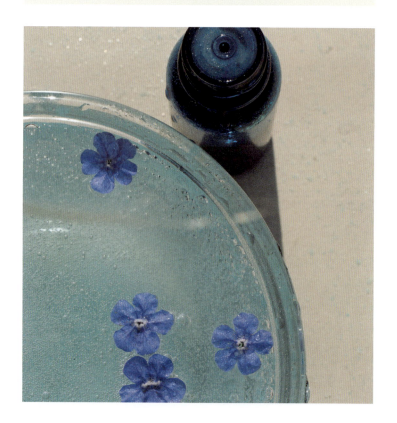

How to Make

- Measure out the sea salt crystals into a big mixing bowl

- Add the liquid pigment

- Stir the mixture thoroughly until the pigment is evenly distributed

- Add the drops of essential oil and stir in well

- Add the bicarbonate of soda and citric acid

- Add any dried botanicals

- Mix everything together gently

- Spoon into decorative glass jars

- Lid and label

How to Use
(with botanicals)

Run a warm bath, pour the mixture into a fine gauze bag or muslin square and tie securely. Immerse the bag in the warm water and allow the salts to fizz and disperse.

How to Use
(without botanicals)

Pour the salts directly into a warm bath and enjoy!

Storage

Fizzing salts may be stored in an airtight jar for several years.

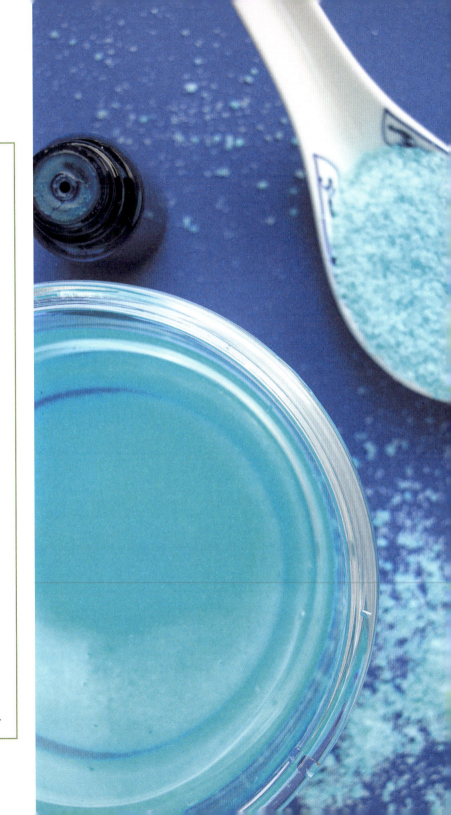

AN EXTRACT FROM
EDINBURGH PHARMACOPOEIA
(1699)

SIMPLE DISTILLED WATERS
(*AQUAE STILLATITIAE SIMPLICES*)

Remedies referred to as *Aquae stillatitiae* (distilled waters) abound in the pages of early herbals – never more so than those that date from around the 17th century – and herbology's beloved edition of Culpeper is no exception. Distillates are to be found equally amongst the old receipts (or recipe books) of the 'gentlewomen' of that time and the first edition of the *Edinburgh Pharmacopoeia* has more than its fair share of meticulously compiled pages dedicated to this gentle art.

An extensive variety of *Materia medica* (not just the purely botanical) would be used as the principal ingredients of these medicinal distillates. The distillate section of the *Edinburgh Pharmacopoeia* includes many 'sweet scented herbs and flowers' which would be found to be most bountiful in the physic garden during the early and later summer months, such as angelica, mugwort, rue, parsley, mint, nettle, meadowsweet, fennel, eyebright, raspberries, blueberries, strawberries, black cherries, and the flowers of chamomile, roses, lime trees, elders, beans and water-lily. The most intriguing distillate ingredient listed in the *Edinburgh Pharmacopoeia* of 1699 has to be frogspawn, but no directions for preparation are provided – just as well perhaps, as we might have felt obliged to include that one in the spring chapter!

The simple distillate recipes noted in the *Edinburgh Pharmacopoeia* are waters of (bitter) oranges, waters of cinnamon (with and without wine) and Queen of Hungary water. These 'simple waters'

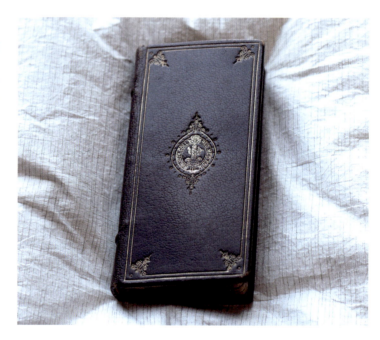

are followed by distillates referred to as *Aquae compositae* or 'compound waters', and include 'alexiterial milk water' (*Aqua lactis alexiteria*) – *alexterial* being an antidote remedy distilled from handfuls of milk thistle leaves and other (hepato-restorative) therapeutic greens; 'hysteric water' (*Aqua hysterica*), which requires a couple of pounds of the poisonous bryony root (*Bryonia dioica*) so definitely not recommended for home use, and 'treacle water' (*Aqua theriacalis*), which sounds comparatively benign and incorporates a couple of the legendary poison antidote *theriaca* (treacles) amongst its other ingredients.

WATER OF (BITTER) ORANGES (*AQUA AURANTIORUM*)

'Take: One pound of the zest of freshly peeled oranges

Six pints of best Spirit of Wine (ethyl alcohol)

Macerate for a couple of days in a well closed vessel, then distil by Alembic in hot sand (i.e. a sand bath) according to standard practice.'

The *Edinburgh Pharmacopoeia* recommends that for the purposes of distillation all the botanicals used are best moderately warmed:

Moistened with a small quantity of spring water; but those that are to be moistened with the same amount of water with a little slat of tartar. Then put them in a small cask, or glazed earthenware jar, tightly stopped and closed from the air, and then let them stand in a temperate place until they become lukewarm. Then immediately let them be distilled, according to standard practice by a Vesica (common still). Let herbs and flowers that are cold, gathered fresh on a fair day, be distilled without any preparation. To those that are dry you may add a greater amount of water, to those that re moist, less.

Author's note: *The above has been kindly translated by Robert Mill, Royal Botanic Garden Edinburgh Research Associate, from the original Latin text of the first edition of* Edinburgh Pharmacopoeia *(1699).*

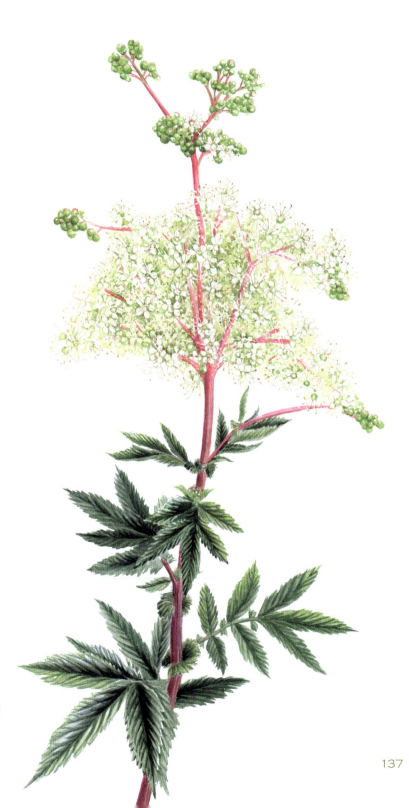

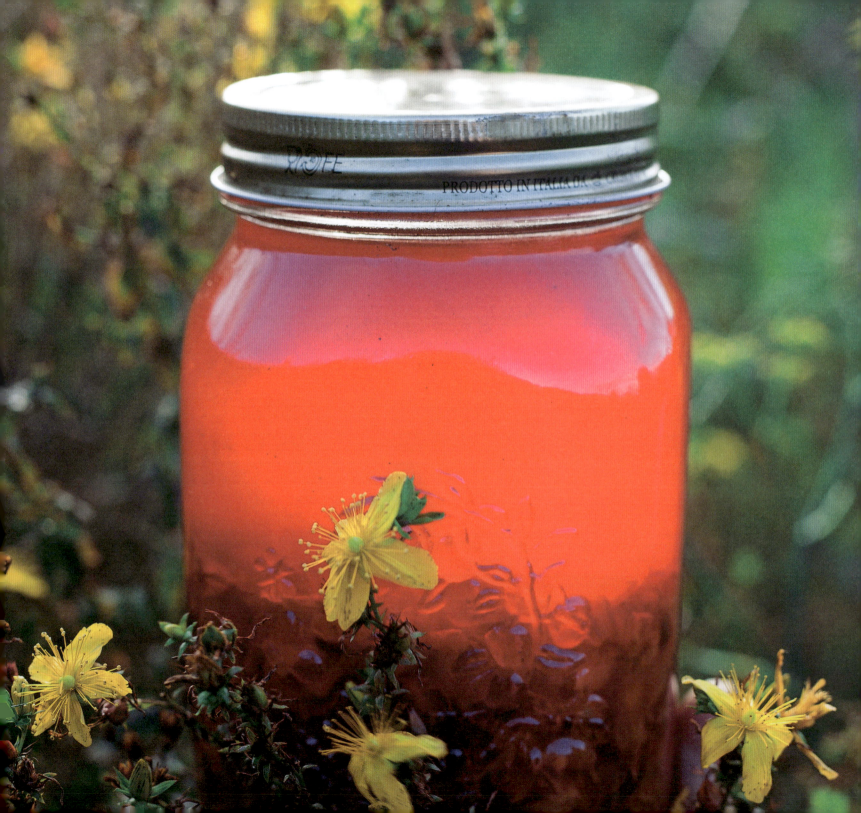

HYPERICUM PERFORATUM

To choose just one flower that represents the summer or might even be considered a 'herb of the sun' from Sutherland's *Hortus Medicus Edinburgensis* (1683) is really an impossibility and every (physic) gardener since his day and every current herbologist will have their favourites.

However, it is perhaps the common St John's wort (*Hypericum perforatum*) that encapsulates so much of what the summer really represents within the herbology physic garden calendar that truly sets it apart from all the other botanicals.

Sutherland lists five different species being grown in the original Edinburgh Physic Garden during the late 17th century, including a tree or shrub St John's wort, a woolly St John's wort and a creeping St John's wort – but only the *Hypericum vulgare* is noted as being medicinal. Its abundance of yellow flowers around midsummer (or a little later) is a seasonal feature within the herbology herb beds. Noted in Culpeper as being under the dominion of the sun it's tempting to wonder if it might have been similarly appreciated in Sutherland's day? We like to think so.

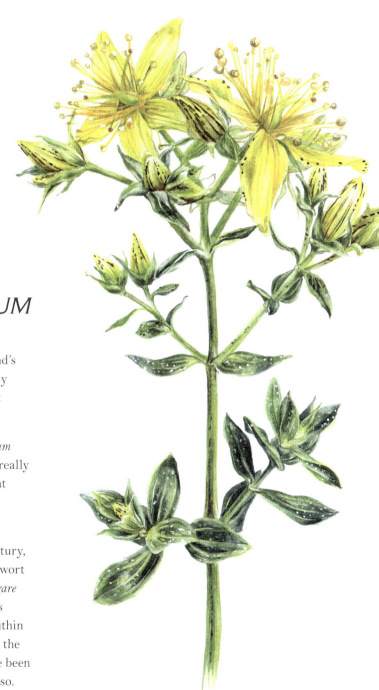

139

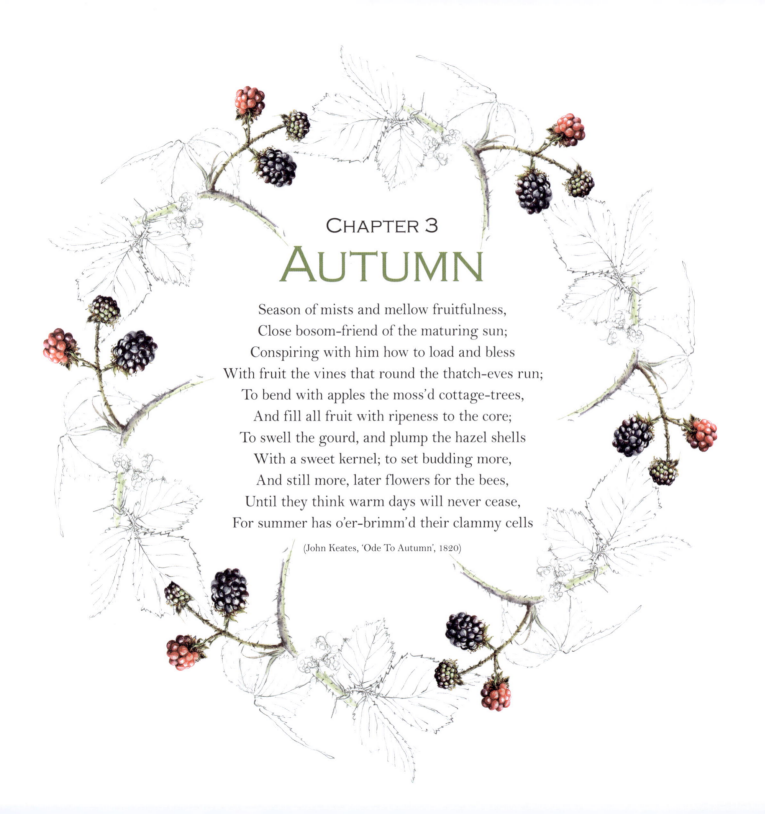

CHAPTER 3
AUTUMN

Season of mists and mellow fruitfulness,
Close bosom-friend of the maturing sun;
Conspiring with him how to load and bless
With fruit the vines that round the thatch-eves run;
To bend with apples the moss'd cottage-trees,
And fill all fruit with ripeness to the core;
To swell the gourd, and plump the hazel shells
With a sweet kernel; to set budding more,
And still more, later flowers for the bees,
Until they think warm days will never cease,
For summer has o'er-brimm'd their clammy cells

(John Keates, 'Ode To Autumn', 1820)

For a moment in September the days seem to hang like golden threads; time distilled from the summer, full of the lingering vestiges of warm sun and ever-burgeoning gardens.

The swifts and swallows, so vociferous in their earlier cable gatherings, have departed for warmer climes and a soft haze shimmers in the mellowed light that now lances ever lower across lawns and walks. A gentle chill descends at twilight, as something almost imperceptible turns in the air and autumn steals upon us.

Truly, this must be one of the most beautiful months in the gardener's calendar…

Heavily dewed lawns reveal the deep, damp prints of all who pass upon them; while garden paths, crisscrossed with the silver trails of snails, make traceable the full extent of their nocturnal meanderings.

Apples and other orchard fruits such as plums and damsons ripen exuberantly on the bough, late roses and other blooms unfurl themselves with the blousy abandon of a last hurrah, and the fragrant balsam-like flowers of shrubs such as *Escallonia* are yet busy with the tireless attentions of their ever-dutiful honeybees.

The drupes of clustered, juicy, purple-staining fruits are irresistible to blackberry pickers; similarly the jewel-like glow of hips and haws, raspberries, blackcurrants and sea buckthorn, or the dusky allure of the gin-making sloes – precious ingredients for herbology's early autumn green pharmacy.

Fiery sunsets fade into dream-like dusks and nature now seems at her most resplendent, with every shade of burnished amber, crimson and all the shimmering yellow-golds as her adornment – at least until the wilder winds roar in! One of the simplest of childhood pleasures is rekindled at the sight of all the gleaming conkers bursting from their spiny cases and peppering the ground beneath the arching boughs of chestnut trees.

From late September onwards, the evocative calls of the incoming wild Canada geese may be heard honking as they wing by overhead. These courageous travellers, navigators of a thousand miles, are almost at their journey's end, returning every year as they do to overwinter in their favourite feeding grounds; the first strains of their audible flight paths being one of the most emotive markers for the change of season.

The pagan fire festival of Samhain, which falls at the end of October, marks the shortening hours of sunlight and the true onset of the darker months of the year. As the nights draw in and the light of the sun diminishes, All Hallows' Eve lanterns and bonfire piles are lit and it does indeed feel, as so often has been said, that only the thinnest of veils now separates our own world from that of the spirit realms and afterlife.

It is time now to draw one year to its close and attune ourselves to the natural energies returning to the earth and the prevailing, almost tangible power of the darkness.

The stars and distant galaxies are at their very brightest in these darker nights of late autumn and early winter, and the beaver full moon of November is resplendent as it follows its own shimmering orbit through this celestial infinity, just as it has done for a billion years.

PHYSIC GARDEN DIARY

THINGS TO DO IN THE PHYSIC GARDEN

The humblest of harvests, hedgerow gleanings or a final herb bed gathering delight the soul in autumn, and the tantalising promises of earlier seasons seem more than fulfilled. This is indeed the time of nature's bounty.

Now is the time to dig up some of the finest medicinal roots, as the earth ruminates and takes back unto itself all that is too fragile to be borne above ground during these colder times, and while the worms – silent collaborators of soil-sustaining decomposition – draw the fallen leaf litter slowly down into their loamy holes.

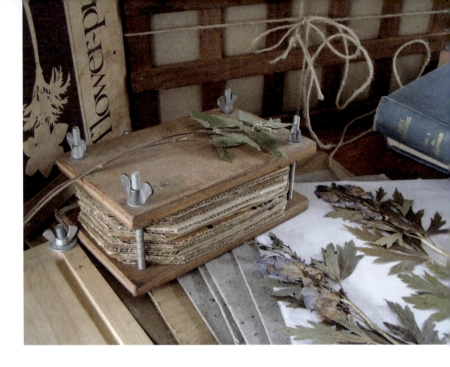

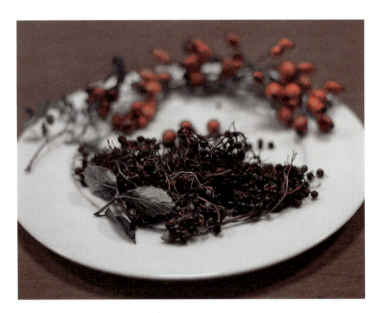

Herb beds may be cleared of all but the hardiest of perennials, or those that bear seeds for the birds and other small foragers, or for next year's garden sowings. And so, we prune and cut back shrubberies, nurture compost piles and bury our manure-filled horns – a ritual we practise every year with our herbology students at the Garden, burying it in one of our herb beds for the duration of winter, to be unearthed in spring and dispersed (rather like a tonic) over the earth that sustains our medicinal botanicals.

Evelyn's September entry in the *Kalendarium Hortense* begins with his recommendation to: 'Gather now if ripe your Winter Fruits, as Apples, Pears, Plums, &c to prevent their falling by the great winds: Also gather your wind falls from day to day: do this work in dry weather.'

How appealing is that promise of 'winter fruits' – the gathering of which must be among the most satisfying for any gardener (or those who indulge in a small share of gleanings from the wild).

But this is just the beginning of the autumnal delights in a 17th-century gardener's calendar of things to do:

I. 'No longer now defer the taking of your Bees,' says Evelyn (clearly a little vexed by all the Vespidae visitors to his garden). With the cider making in full flow, he writes, 'Continue still your hostility against wasps, and other robbing insects!'

It is so easy to imagine in the increasingly drowsy days of late September, the intoxicating brews of fermenting apples and the somewhat fervid buzzings of the drunken wasps! Evelyn then writes:

II. Now is also the time to turn to your flower beds. Gather autumnal flowers 'to prevent sudden gusts which will also prostrate all that you have so industriously rais'd'

III. Transplant 'fibrous plants' such as chamomile, violets and primroses

IV. 'About Michaelmas (sooner, or later, as the Season directs) the weather fair, and by no means foggy, retire your choice greens, and rarest plants (being dry) … into your Conservatory; ordering them with fresh mould as you were taught in May'

With 'the cold now advancing' Evelyn recommends:

V. 'Set such plants as will not endure the warm indoors "into the earth".' Their pots should be placed a couple of inches lower than the surface of the bed they are being moved to, which should be of a southern exposure

VI. 'Then cover them with glasses, having cloath'd them first with Sweet & dry Moss; but upon all warm and benign & emissions of the Sun, and Sweet showers, giving them air, by taking off all that covers them'

VII. Of the many flowers Evelyn notes as being still in their 'prime or yet lasting' includes: candy tufts, poppies of all colours, passion flowers, myrtles, musk rose and Persian autumnal narcissus

In October, we are told to undertake the following tasks:

VIII. 'Trench Ground for Orcharding' and the kitchen garden 'to lie for a Winter mellowing'

IX. Now is the time for 'laying bare the Roots of old unthriving, or hasty blooming trees'

X. With a moon now 'decreasing', Evelyn recommends gathering winter fruits and to 'take heed of bruising'

XI. Cut and prune roses and bury 'all sorts of bulbous roots'

XII. And perhaps most nurturing for the soul of all, he reminds us to 'make Winter Cider'!

By the time November comes in his *Kalendarium*, Evelyn urges that we:

XIII. 'Lose no time, hard Frosts come on apace'

XIV. These last moments in which one might reasonably complete the year's gardening tasks are when to 'carry compost out of your Melon ground or turn, and mingle it with the earth, and lay it in Ridges ready for the Spring'

XV. Sow and set early beans and peas and gather the last of the orchard fruits

XVI. 'Cover your peeping Ranunculus' – indeed, cover peeping everything!

XVII. Around the middle of this month (or sooner, if weather requires), enclose your tender plants 'secluding all entrance of cold, and especially sharp winds; and if the plants become exceeding dry, and that it do not actually freeze, refresh them sparingly with qualified water, mingled with a little sheeps, or Cow-dung'

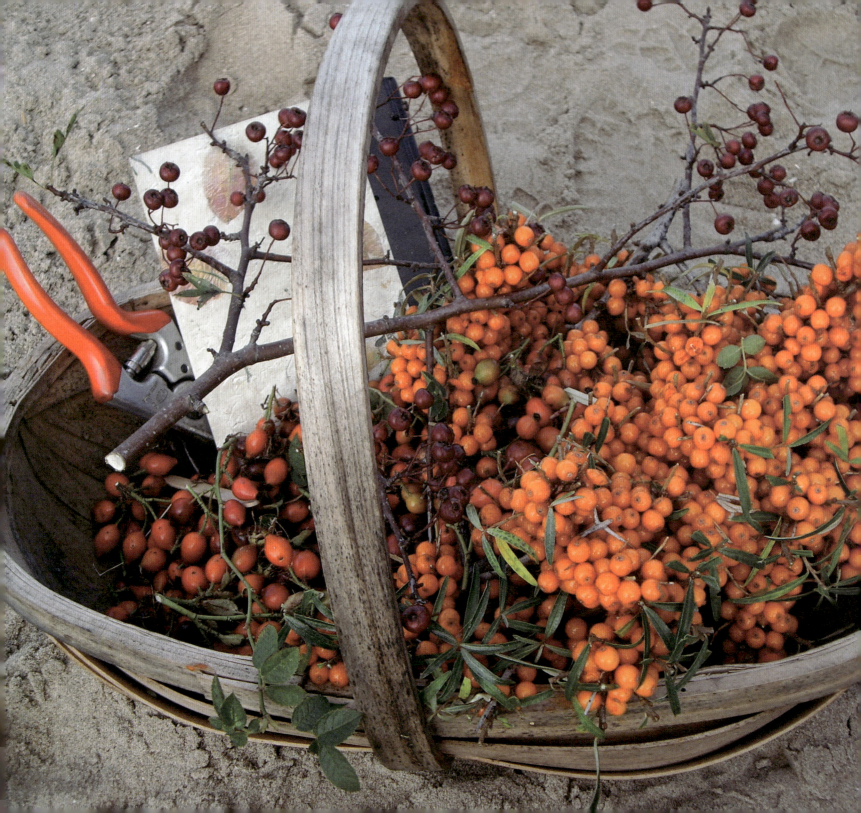

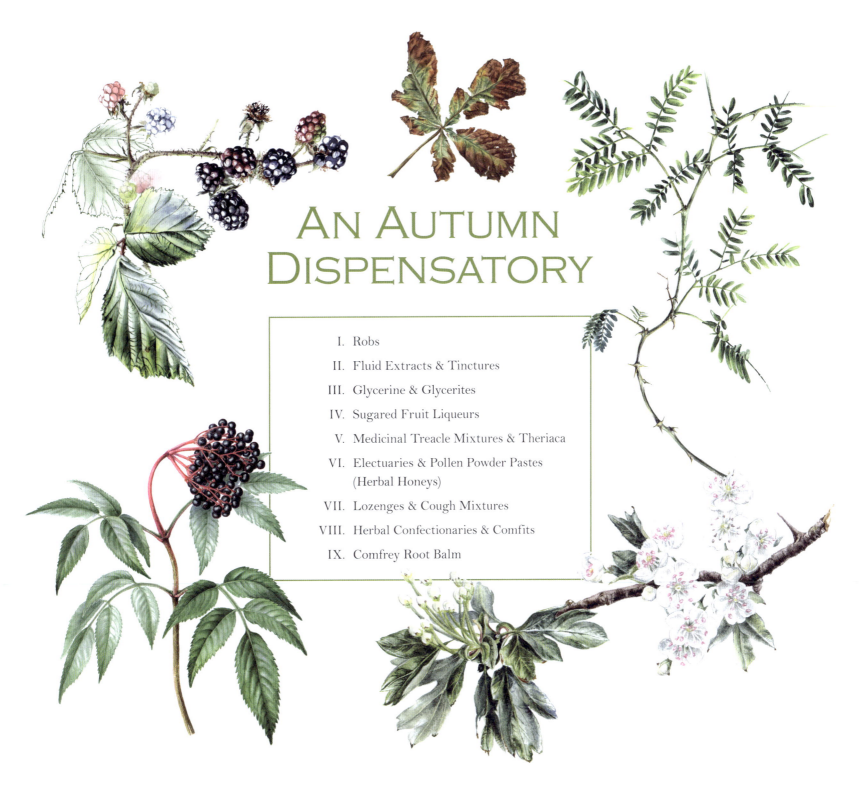

An Autumn Dispensatory

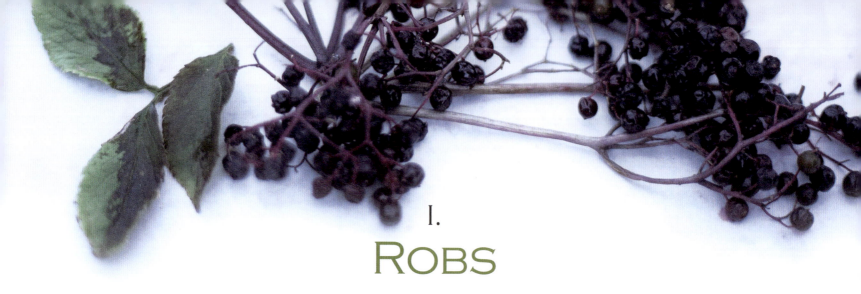

I.

ROBS

WHAT ARE ROBS?

'Robs' are thick medicinal syrups, and one of our oldest and most enduring (and endearing) herbal remedies. Recipes for robs appeared everywhere during the 17th century, beginning with 'elderberry rob', the 'official' pharmacopoeia favourite. In fact, robs or 'musts' (wines that are boiled until thick) noted alongside the more familiar elderberry in the first edition of the *Edinburgh Pharmacopoeia* (1699) include one for 'barberry' (*Berberis*) fruits, another for juniper berries (which makes no mention of sugar being added) and one for a currant rob, which is made to the traditional (and sugary) recipe that follows – and sounds rather good! Contemporary rob recipes follow much the same methodology, depending on whether you prefer sugar or honey.

ELDERBERRY ROB

It would seem that the elderberry rob – traditionally made from the expressed juice of fresh elderberries, simmered with spices and thickened with either sugar or honey – is perhaps the best loved of all the robs. Like many other fruit robs, the elderberry rob would be prepared in the late summer and early autumn

for use throughout the chillier times of winter. Many of the old herbal dispensaries used to sell hot toddy-like measures to 'warm the heart' and ward off the season's most prevalent ills because these robs were, and still are, considered by far the most excellent remedies for any type of cold or influenza.

Elderberries are full of antioxidant, antiviral and immune-boosting flavonoid compounds, including rutin, purple black anthocyanidin pigments, tannins and vitamin C. They are also high in viburnic acid, which gives elderberry the diaphoretic, eliminative and thereby detoxifying effect that it is so well-recognised for. An all-round fantastically efficacious remedy to help the body fight against infections.

Author's note: *The word 'rob' may have some old root connections to another beverage known as a 'shrub', itself derived from the Arabic 'sharaba', which has been used to denote, among other things, a syrup. Shrubs were developed in England during the 15th century and were a form of revitalising medicine, made from the juice of fruit, with sugar and other ingredients – usually an alcohol such as brandy – so they very closely resembled a liqueur. The robs of our herbals are notably alcohol-free, but they would make an excellent cocktail!*

TRADITIONAL ELDERBERRY ROB RECIPE

INGREDIENTS
(given in the old imperial pounds and ounces)

5lb fresh ripe, crushed elderberries

1lb loaf sugar (sugar lumps)

HOW TO MAKE

- Put the elderberries in a heavy pot
- Add the loaf sugar
- Simmer gently until the sugar has dissolved and the juice has reduced to the thickness of honey
- Pour into sterilised jars, lid and label

HOW TO TAKE

A couple of tablespoonfuls mixed in a glass of hot water to be taken at night. It promotes perspiration and is demulcent and soothing to the chest.

STORAGE

Store in a cool, dark place for use in the winter.

Author's note: *Only ripe black, cooked elderberries should be used in herbal remedies as they are toxic if eaten raw*

CONTEMPORARY (SPICED) ELDERBERRY ROB RECIPE

INGREDIENTS

300ml elderberry juice extract

150g raw cane sugar or 150ml organic honey

OPTIONAL INGREDIENTS

Stick of cinnamon

A few cloves

Several star anise or a pinch of ginger root powder

A slice of lemon

HOW TO MAKE

- Warm the elderberry juice extract gently in a heavy-bottomed pan, together with the sugar or honey
- Add the spices or a slice of lemon to the mixture and simmer gently for around 30 minutes, stirring regularly
- Once the sugar or honey has dissolved, pour into sterilised jars, lid and label

HOW TO TAKE

A teaspoonful, as required (up to three times a day), or stir a teaspoonful into hot water and drink.

STORAGE

Store in the fridge and use within a couple of months.

SUGAR-FREE ELDERBERRY ROB RECIPE

INGREDIENTS

A couple of handfuls of elderberries

Spices to taste: try cinnamon, cloves, star anise, cardamom or ginger

A little water (a cupful or so)

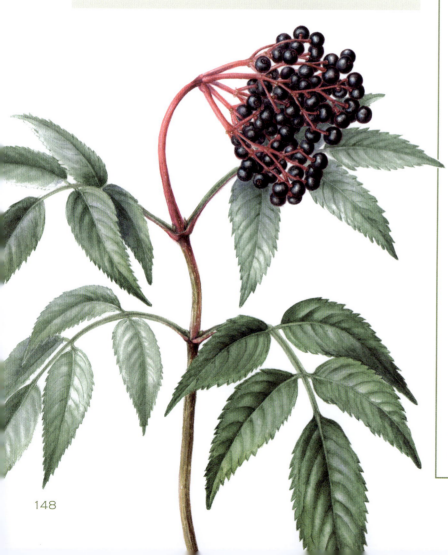

HOW TO MAKE

- Begin by making a decoction of the elderberries by removing the ripe berries from their stalks, rinsing in cold water and placing in a heavy-bottomed pot with a little cold water and spices of your choice

- Lid the pot, and bring the mixture to a gentle simmer for a few minutes

- Squash the berries with a wooden spoon or the end of a rolling pin to express the juice

- Simmer with the lid on, very gently, for a further 30 minutes

- Next, strain the remnant berries and spices from the decocted liquid and return the decoction to the pot

- Resume the simmer (uncovered this time) on a very low heat

- Once the liquid has reduced by half or is the thickness of molasses, your rob is ready

- Pour the liquid into sterilised wide-mouthed jars (robs, rather like herbal honeys can solidify like jam as they cool and can therefore be tricky to get out of bottles)

HOW TO TAKE

Around 10ml, three times a day. Alternatively, half a small cup may be warmed gently and sipped before sleep, perhaps with a little local honey melted in.

STORAGE

Store in the fridge and consume within one week or freeze in smaller amounts until required.

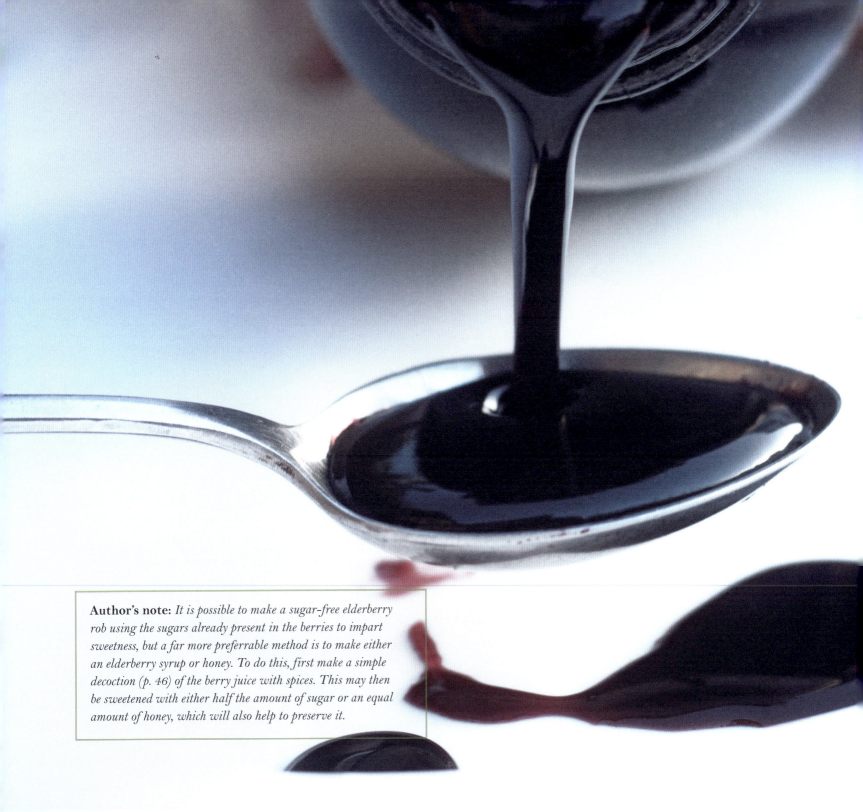

Author's note: *It is possible to make a sugar-free elderberry rob using the sugars already present in the berries to impart sweetness, but a far more preferrable method is to make either an elderberry syrup or honey. To do this, first make a simple decoction (p. 46) of the berry juice with spices. This may then be sweetened with either half the amount of sugar or an equal amount of honey, which will also help to preserve it.*

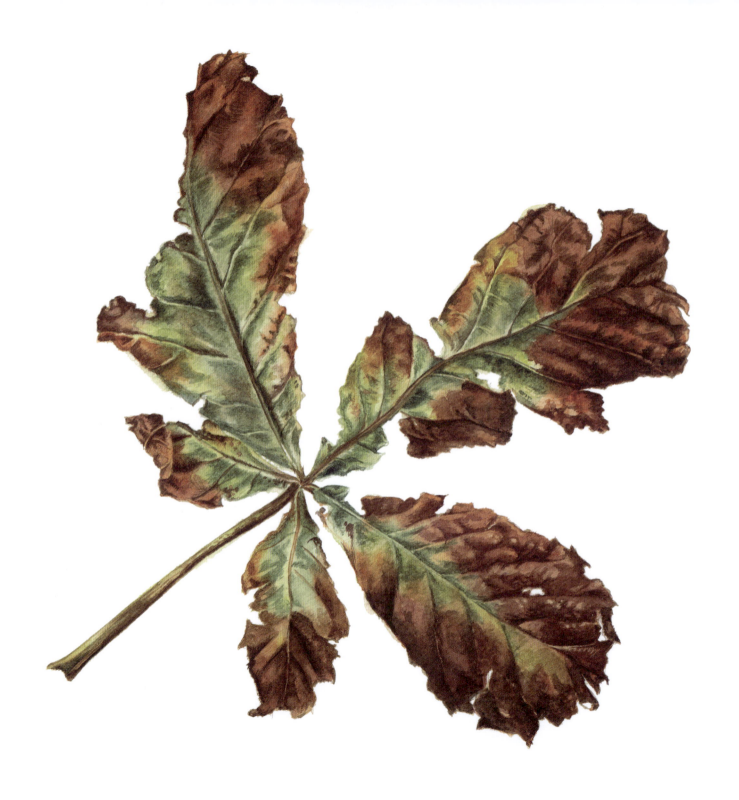

II.

FLUID
EXTRACTS &
TINCTURES

There is nothing quite so pleasurable during the darkening days of autumn than to be ensconced in the library, turning the hallowed and sepia-tinted pages of one of the older editions of Culpeper's *Complete Herbal* (1653), when you happen chance upon something like this:

Tinctura Croci (Tincture of Saffron)

Take two drams of Saffron, eight ounces of Treacle water, digest them six days, then strain it.

See the Virtues of Treacle water, and then know that this strengthens the heart something more, and keeps melancholy vapours thence by drinking a spoonful of it every morning.

Such a delightful and simple recipe, it seems, and how tempting it is to contemplate the preparation of this saffron-infused tincture. It sounds the perfect remedy to offset the wistful nostalgia that can steal upon the cheeriest of souls with the onset of autumn.

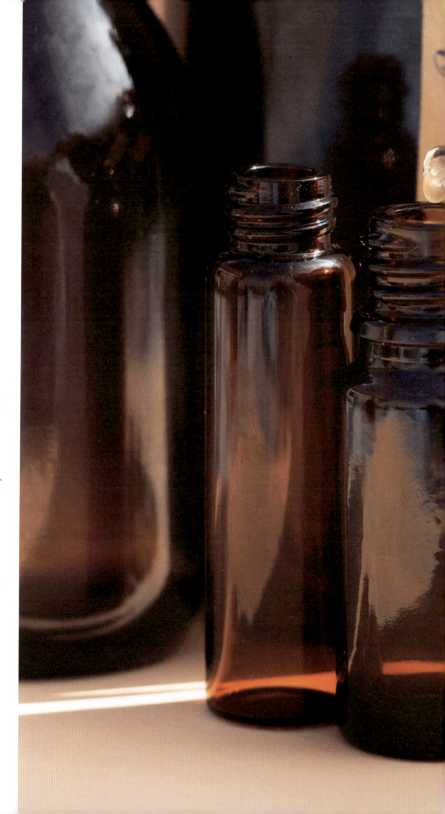

WHAT ARE TINCTURES?

Quite simply, tinctures are botanically infused solutions of pure ethyl alcohol and water, into which the active constituents of the botanical have been extracted. But unlike liqueurs and herbal and fruit gins, which may be drunk quite freely (and it must be said, far more pleasurably), tinctures are highly concentrated, prepared by and for our herbal dispensaries following recognised (and fairly standardised) formulae – quite far removed from the tinctures of Culpeper's time!

All alcoholic extracts (of whatever form) provide a relatively simple and effective way to hold onto the therapeutic goodness of the botanicals we love way after they have disappeared from our pots, plots or physic gardens.

Depending on which part of a botanical is recommended for use in herbal healing, you may encounter the tinctured alcoholic extracts of root, bud, leaf, fruit, flower, bark, seed, and even resin and pollen in the medical herbalist store.

For the purposes of this book, our tincture recipes follow what is frequently referred to as the 'folk method'. This enables us to make the most of already diluted (with water) vodka as our principle alcohol of choice and therefore avoids much of the often befuddling but necessary mathematical calculations required of the more involved (pharmaceutical grade) formulations that require a licence to make!

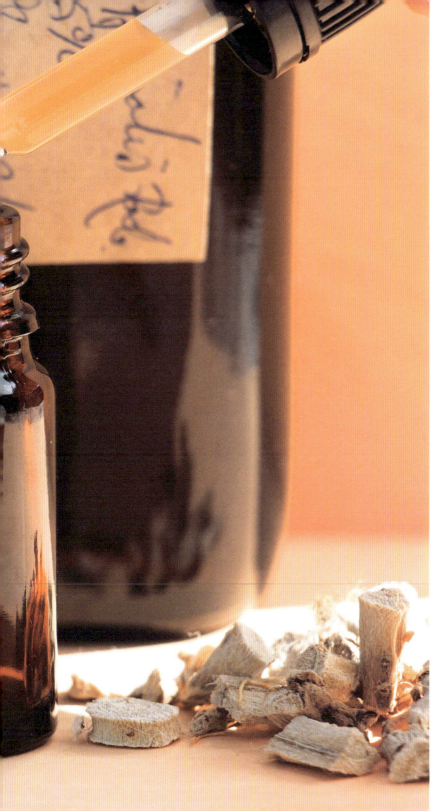

It is generally agreed among most herbalists that 40%-strength alcohol is sufficient to extract a good balance of the water- and alcohol-soluble constituents from most medicinal botanicals. So, this is what is recommend for use here. It is good to be aware of the strength of the extract you are making – the ratios are always given weight to volume, e.g. 1g botanical to 5ml alcohol, which may be written as 1:5. This is a good ratio generally, but you could experiment with either a stronger 1:3 or weaker 1:10. A fluid extract is the most concentrated form of tincture – it is made from equal parts of herb to alcohol and is referred to as a '1 in 1', or more correctly. Please note, a tincture below 18.5% alcohol will go off.

Tinctures are strong medicines and are far more potent, volume for volume, than infusions or decoctions, so always seek advice from a qualified medical herbalist before you begin to make these sorts of remedies at home – especially regarding the appropriate choice of botanical. Please note that tinctured alcoholic extracts are not recommended for children or the very elderly. Instead, try our infusions (p. 45), glycerites (p. 156) or warm herbal milks (p. 48), which are a wonderful bedtime remedy.

Here are a couple of easy-to-follow recipes that should yield some very satisfying tinctures.

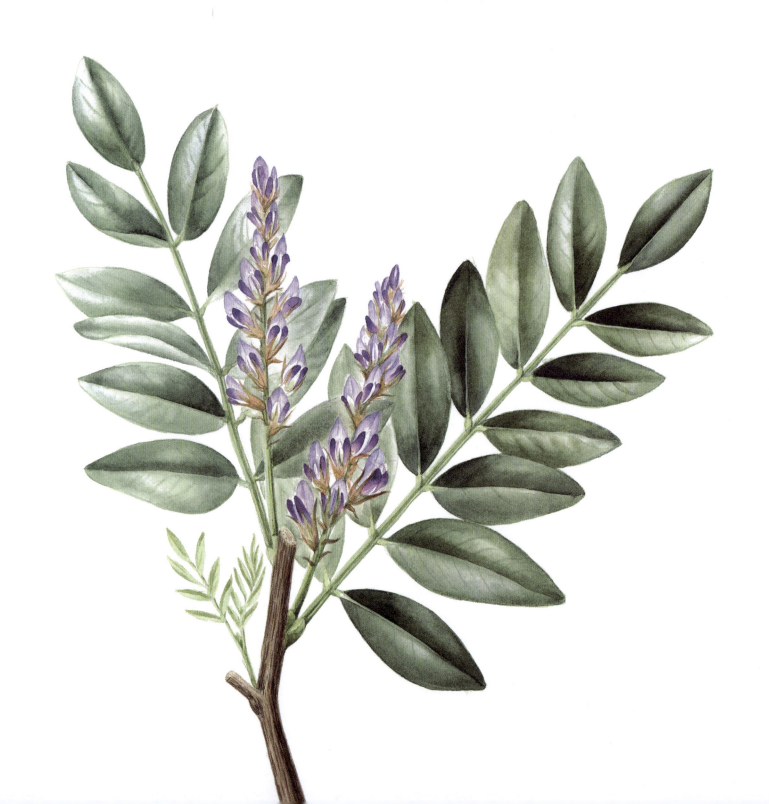

AUTUMNAL ALCOHOLIC EXTRACTS
RECIPE

INGREDIENTS FOR
DRIED BOTANICAL EXTRACT (1:5)

20g dried medicinal botanical (try echinacea root, bilberry, aniseed, astragalus root, elderberry, liquorice root, blackberry, angelica root, Ceylon cinnamon bark, bitter orange or ginger root)

100ml 40% vodka (or alternative with no lower than 25% strength – the minimum required for this recipe)

INGREDIENTS FOR
FRESH BOTANICAL EXTRACT (1:3)

100g fresh medicinal botanical
(as opposite, but freshly gathered)

300ml 40% vodka
(be aware that fresh botanicals
may hold as much as 80% water,
which dilutes the strength of the alcohol)

HOW TO MAKE

- If you're using dried botanicals, cut them into small pieces or grind to a powder

- If you're using fresh botanicals, chop and gently crush

- Place the pieces or powder into a glass jar with a tight screw-top lid

- Pour the alcohol onto the botanical and seal the jar well

- Shake vigorously

- Store the jar in a warm, dark place for a fortnight, shaking it thoroughly several times a day

- Once ready, strain out the bulk of the liquid extract

- Express any remaining extract through a muslin square over a bowl or jug

- Pour the tincture into a dark amber glass bottle

- Date, lid and label

HOW TO TAKE

One teaspoon diluted in a little water or fruit juice, three times a day. Please check the correct dosage of botanicals in one of the recommended herbals listed at the back of this book (p. 241). Be aware of possible contraindications.

STORAGE

Tinctures made from dried botanical ingredients may be stored for up to three years in a cool, dark place, but ideally consume within one year of making.

Author's note: *The left-over marc (or exhausted botanical) from either fresh or dried botanical tincture-making is an excellent compost material.*

III.
GLYCERINE &
GLYCERITES

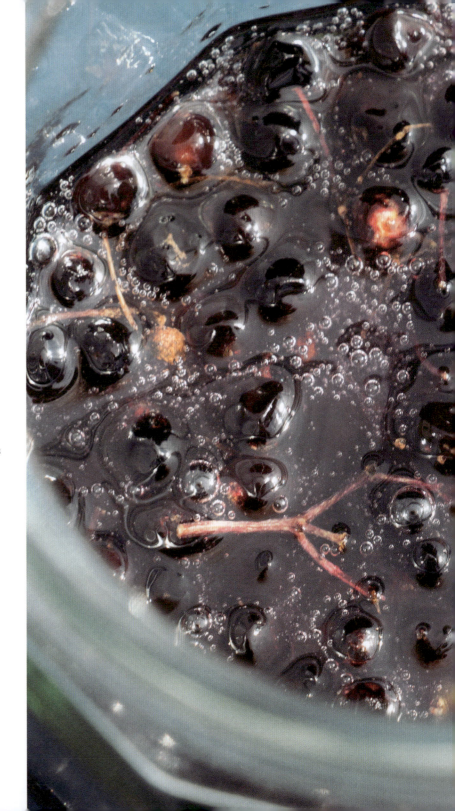

A glycerite is a non-alcoholic remedy made from botanicals that have been extracted into either a purely glycerine- or glycerine-water-based solution.

Glycerine itself is a clear, sticky, very sweet demulcent, emollient and hygroscopic liquid, extracted from fats and oils – it has different sources. It is the organic vegetable, glycerine, that is preferred in herbal medicine making. Glycerine is often used by herbalists to prevent phlobatannins (condensed tannins including anthocyanidins), gums and mucilage from forming precipitates in tinctured alcoholic extracts, which they tend to do.

Here are some formulae for their preparation. As before, we recommend that only small sample measures are prepared initially, but however much you make, you need to make sure that your glycerine concentration is sufficient to preserve it.

We recommend one part water to three parts glycerine for dried botanical ingredients (or a minimum of 55%) and 100% pure glycerine for fresh botanical ingredients.

Author's note: *Glycerine, rather like honey, naturally attracts moisture. The high water content of fresh botanicals will quickly dilute it – hence the 100% pure glycerine requirement for these.*

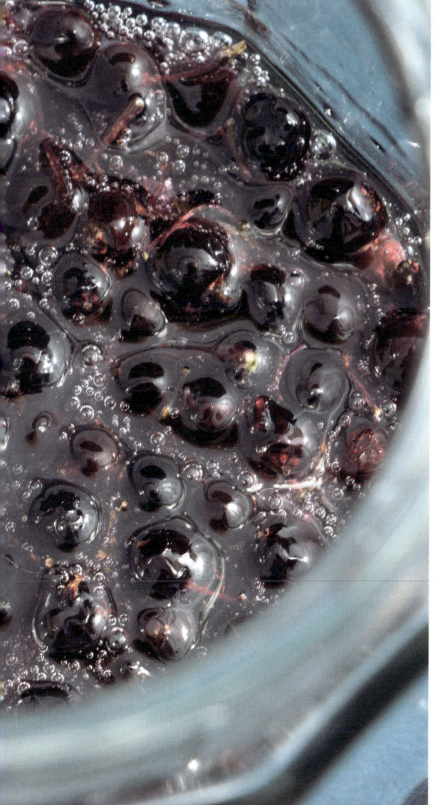

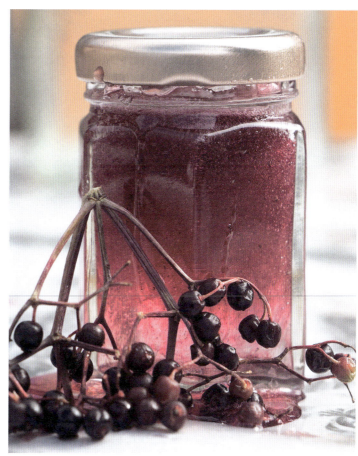

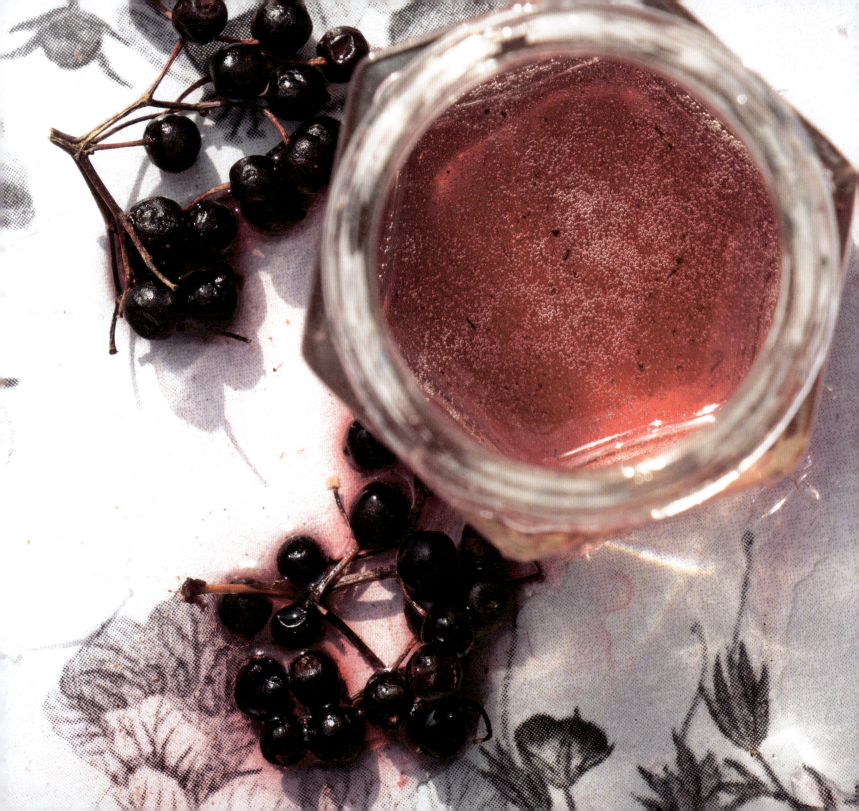

GLYCERITE
RECIPE

INGREDIENTS FOR
DRIED BOTANICAL GLYCERITE

120ml glycerine

80ml cold distilled water

50g dried and ground botanical pieces (try echinacea root, bilberry, aniseed, astragalus root, elderberry, liquorice root, blackberry, angelica root, Ceylon cinnamon bark, bitter orange or ginger root)

INGREDIENTS FOR
FRESH BOTANICAL GLYCERITE

50g fresh botanical (see those listed on p. 155)

150ml glycerine

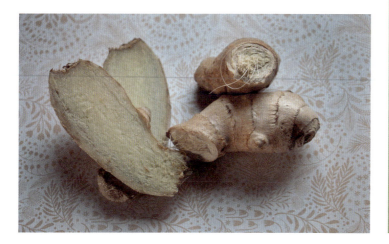

HOW TO MAKE

- Put both the botanical ingredient and the glycerine in a blender and blitz

- Pour into a small enough jar so that it is full with minimal air space

- Lid the jar and allow to infuse for a fortnight – agitate the jar frequently during this time

- Strain and squeeze out the resultant glycerite liquid from the remaining botanical through a piece of muslin

- Pour into amber glass bottles

HOW TO TAKE

Half a teaspoon (ten drops), three times a day, in a little water.

STORAGE

Store in a cool, dark place for up to a year.

Author's note: *A little vitamin C, citric acid powder or lemon juice can be added as a final preparation to help preserve these mixtures, raise their immune-boosting potential and dissipate some of the sweetness.*

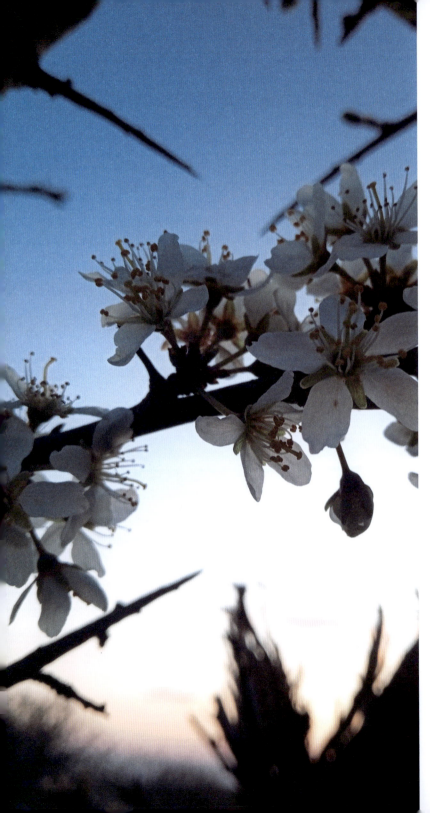

IV.
SUGARED FRUIT LIQUEURS

Liqueurs are made from alcoholic spirits infused with the flavours of fruits, herbs and spices that have been extracted into them. They're un-aged, beyond the period required for their flavours to mingle and meld. A true liqueur should be drunk neat and in relatively small quantities – one liqueur glassful at a time!

Beautifully coloured translucent liqueurs made from late summer and early autumn fruits warm the heart and lift the spirits on chilly, dark winter nights – or indeed, whenever one feels the need for a little pick-me-up! Try lingering winter liqueurs on a summer evening, poured over ice.

Whenever you enjoy them, now is the time to make fruit liqueurs in eager readiness for Yuletide, Christmas and all the other such festivities.

A good fruit liqueur is smooth and quite heavily sweetened with dissolved sugar (the word 'liqueur' is derived from the Latin *liquifacere*, which means 'to dissolve'). Their syrup-like solution softens some of the bitterness that might otherwise be imparted from sour fruits. Liqueurs are naturally rich in medicinal compounds and originated as herbal medicines – many recipes for them are hundreds of years old. Some, like Chartreuse, were and still are prepared by monks.

The recipe that follows, given in the old imperial pounds and ounces, has been passed down through my own family and originally used damson fruits and loaf sugar, but a whole variety of tarter fruits could be used, e.g. blackcurrants, redcurrants, rhubarb, sea buckthorn berries, gooseberries, cherries, etc.

Sloe or Damson Gin Recipe

Ingredients
(given in the old imperial pounds and ounces)

1lb 8oz sloes (nicely ripened fruits)

1lb lump sugar (raw cane sugar cubes are recommended)

1 bottle of gin

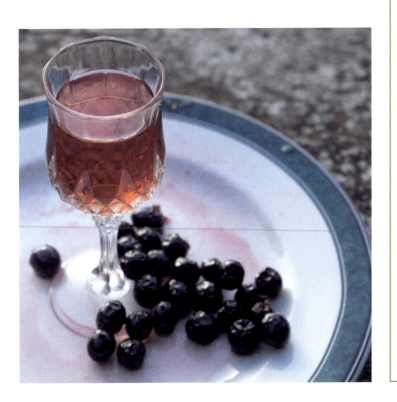

How to Make

- Weigh the sloes and rinse them under cold water
- Tip them all into a bowl and prick over rapidly with a fork (do this several times to help release the juices from each of the fruits)
- Trickle the sloes into a clean glass jar with a screw-top lid
- Add the sugar and pour over the gin
- Lid the jar and shake vigorously
- Allow the gin to infuse for several weeks, swirling the solution around frequently
- Once the sugar has completely dissolved, it's ready

How to Take

One small liqueur glassful as needed, to lift flagging spirits and fatigue.

Storage

These sorts of liqueurs will keep for several years but are probably at their best in their first year.

Author's note: *A 750ml bottle of gin is about right for the weights of sugar and fruit given above. The more gin you use, the more liqueur you will have to enjoy at the end but it will be less sweet and fruity. The recipe lends itself to being adapted, so have a little creative fun with it.*

V.

MEDICINAL TREACLE MIXTURES & THERIACA

Theriaca, or treacle, was one of several different names given to a most extraordinary collection of medicinal mixtures whose original recipes (under the various names of *mithridate, mithridatium, mithridatum* or *mithridaticum*), despite having their origins in antiquity, are very far from lost to it. The fabled reputation of theriaca itself (an antidote to every kind of poison, particularly those from the bites of venomous beasts) peaked on the continent during the Renaissance and remained there until it was apparently last seen being brewed up in Venice in the late 1700s – and then it faded from medicinal use.

It was the Venice treacle that was the most famous and expensive theriaca of them all. This 'treacle' was one of the most complex and highly sought-after medicines ever compounded. At the height of its popularity, some formulations listed over five dozen different ingredients – many of which were considered extremely exotic and hard to come by, increasing not only the desire for the finished mixture but also its value.

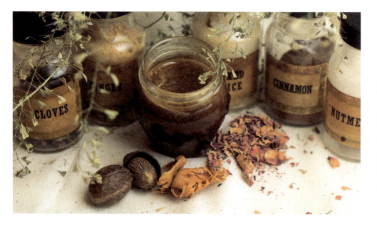

Originally prepared from a myriad of aromatic botanicals, spices, roots, balsams, resins and gums that were sought from the four corners of the world, it was also known to incorporate the dried blood or flesh of lizards or vipers in its later manifestations. 'Castoreum', the excretion from the caster sacs of beavers (or the castor sacs themselves) and the wonderfully named 'malabathrum' (a cinnamon leaf that originates from the Himalayas and was used to flavour wines in the ancient world) were frequently recognised ingredients.

All of these ingredients (as an amalgamation of simples into just one remedy) were bound together in a honey base, so theriaca was effectively a herbal honey. Indeed, the name 'molasses' comes from the Portuguese word *melaço*, which is derived from the Latin *mel*, meaning honey.

Over time the pharmacological meaning associated with treacle faded. Around the 17th century in England, the word itself took on its more contemporary meaning that we now more readily recognise as the dark, sticky sweetener in a tin, while mithridate came to refer to any generally all-purpose antidote.

The following theriaca recipe is handed down by kind permission of a former Royal Botanic Garden Edinburgh Herbology Certificate group, who are happy to share it in the hope that it might lead to even more delicious formulations of this sort. Arguably, they believe that golden syrup makes the yummiest theriaca by far. Whatever the deliciously viscous base ingredient – whether treacle, molasses or honey – the end mixture is bound to be extraordinarily good, probably solid and very sweet….

A Jolly Good Theriaca Recipe

Ingredients

250ml golden syrup

2 tsp dried rosebuds, ground to fine powder

1 tsp black peppercorns, ground to fine powder

½ tsp dried ginger root powder

½ tsp cardamom green seed, ground to fine powder

½ tsp cinnamon dried bark powder

How to Make

- Measure out your chosen 'base' (honey or one of the treacles)
- Pour directly into a pot or bain-marie and place on the hob
- Warm through thoroughly
- Add the selected dried and powdered ingredients
- Mix in thoroughly, using a wooden spoon
- Adjust to taste
- Once ready, pour into sterilised glass jars
- Lid and label

How to Take

As an antidote against all the ills in the world, take one teaspoon as desired or pour over porridge, natural yoghurt or into warm milk.

Storage

This theriaca or 'treacle' will keep for up to a year, if stored in a cool, dark cupboard.

Author's note: *No viper flesh or blood required!*

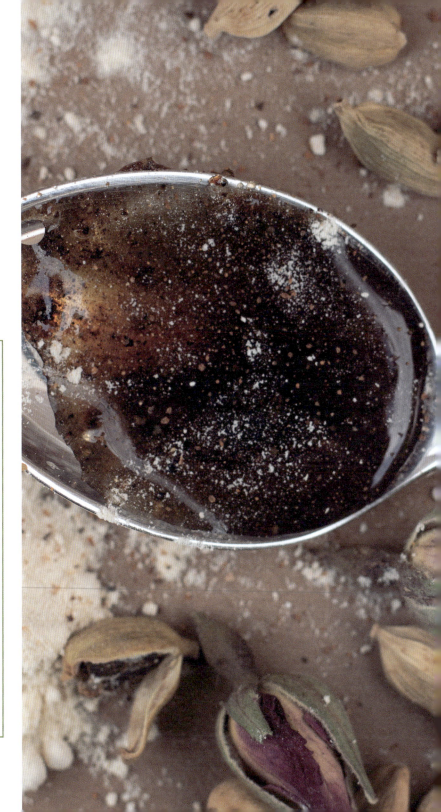

An Extract from Edinburgh Pharmacopoeia (1699)

Theriaca Andromachi (Venice Treacle)

A recipe for Venice treacle called *Theriaca Adromachi* appears in our 17th century *Edinburgh Pharmacopoeia*, and we simply had to include it here. The formulation appears alongside *Theriaca Diatessaron* (common theriac) and an actual recipe for mithridate, *Mithridatum Damocratis – the Mithridate of (Sevilius) Damocrates*, all of which can be found under 'De Antidotis, & Opiatis – Antidotes and Opiates' – this one small book cannot do justice to them all!

The list of ingredients that were included in some of the earliest mithridate and theriaca formulations are quite remarkable and way beyond anything that a herbalist would ever consider pulling together nowadays. Both mithridate and theriaca were recognised as patented medicines within official dispensaries and pharmacopoeias until the 18th century.

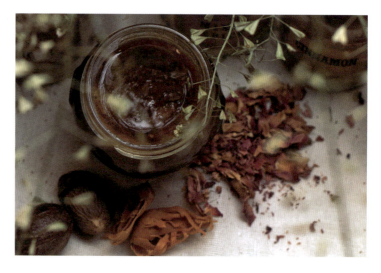

What a piece of work! One can only imagine the effort involved in the acquisition of all these ingredients and how time-consuming it must have been to just measure out the correct amounts for all the individual bits and pieces of *Materia medica* – the actual compounding of it all and mixing everything into a honey base sounds relatively easy! The secret would have been to have everything already prepared – but hasn't that ever been so.

The sheer opulence of this one recipe is quite staggering compared with what one might expect of a contemporary herbal formulation, but of possibly even greater intrigue than this – and almost lost, hiding at the very end of all the other electuaries – is an Edinburgh treacle, *Theriaca Edensis*, discovered in the later 1721 edition of the *Edinburgh Pharmacopoeia*.

Asphalathi scrupulos duos.
Castorei drachmas duas.

In classe sequente singula per se tu-
rantur.

Croci unciam unam.
Boli Armenæ veræ pro Terrâ
    Lemniâ,
Chalcitidis tostæ donec cineri-
    cea fiat, ana unciam semis.
Bituminis Judaici, vel ejus
    defectu, Succini albi
    præparati drachmas
           duas.
Carnis Viperarum exsiccatæ
    uncias tres.

Myrrhæ electæ unciam unam.
Opii Thebaici,
Pulpæ Scyllæ ana uncias tres.
Sagapeni unciam semis.
Thuris Masculi,
Terebinthinæ Chiæ ana drach-
    mas sex.
Styracis Calamitæ.
Succi Acaciæ,
    Hypocystidis ana unci-
    am semis.

                 Succi

Succi Liquiritiæ unciam unam
          semis.

Galbani,
Opoponacis ana drachmas
         duas.
Mastiches Scrupulum unum.
Opobalsami, vel ejus defectu
Olei Nucis Moschatæ per
    expressionem unciam u-
    nam, & drachmas quin-
    que.
Mellis optimi despumati tri-
    plum ad pondus specierum Sicca-
    rum
Vini Canarini generosi q. s. ad
    dissolvendos Succos, & Gummi.
M. fiat s. a. Opiata.

Theriaca Diatesseron.

R. Aristolochiæ Rotundæ,
Gentianæ,
Baccarum Lauri,
Myrrhæ electæ ana uncias du-
    as.
Rob Juniperini.
Mellis optimi despumati ana
        libram unam.

Misce fiat Electuarium s. a.

                 SECTIO

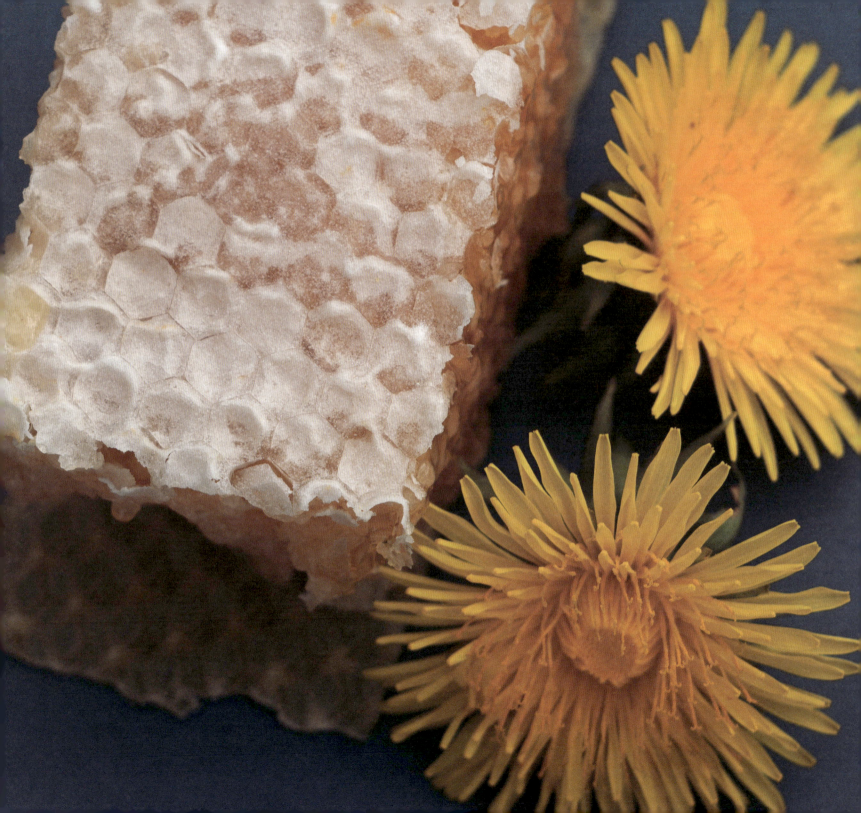

VI.
ELECTUARIES &
POLLEN POWDER PASTES
(HERBAL HONEYS)

Our theriaca recipe leads us nicely to electuaries, or herbal honeys, themselves. Electuaries are among the more familiar remedies found in the herbals and pharmacopoeias of the 17th century – although not all used honey; some were thickened to their consistencies with syrups and/or sugar.

The earliest edition of the *Edinburgh Pharmacopoeia* (1699) has its fair share of electuaries too – some typically more appealing than others. *De Electuariis Purgantibus* translates as 'concerning purging electuaries', but in truth, they date from much earlier and are actually believed to have reached ancient Greece (like all things sweet and good in our herbal pharmacy) from the Arab world.

Honey is one of the most precious ingredients in our *Materia medica* (as indeed are all the gifts we receive from the honeybees) and to use just a little in our recipes seems to imbrue the whole mixture with so much natural goodness. It is a highly demulcent, emollient and nourishing compound that sweetens our herbal remedies in the most healthful and healing of ways.

So, why is honey so good for us? Well, that all comes down to the singularly clever chemistry of the bees themselves, who by their own industry are able to transform the complex sucrose solution of the flower nectars they collect into the simple (and, for us, most easily digestible) sugars, glucose and fructose, of which honey is mostly made. Apart from these super energy-boosting carbohydrates (sugars), honey also holds

many vitamins, minerals, amino acids, enzymes, organic acids, pollen, fragrances and flavour compounds, depending on the botanicals visited by the bees and, to an extent, the geographical locations where they forage for their nectar.

Sometimes referred to as *mel* in herbal and other formularies and recipes, honey is best heated as little as possible during remedy making to preserve its natural therapeutic properties. Unheated honey gradually solidifies (crystallises) over time, and you will discover nearly solid jars of honey languishing in cupboards if they have remained in storage there for any length of time. This solid honey is still perfectly good for remedy making and may be easily liquified again by gentle warming through (in its jar) in the bottom of a very low oven.

Incredibly, solidified honey was found in the tombs of ancient Egypt and was still perfectly edible. The flowers the bees visited all those thousands of years ago were identifiable from the pollen grains it held – isn't that extraordinary!

A simple electuary may be easily made using very finely ground soft herbal powders (see overleaf) or pollen powders mixed with a little honey – once stirred together, this mixture makes a delicious herbal honey or pollen powder paste.

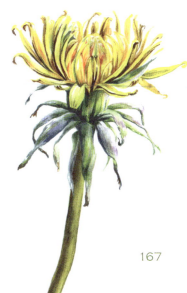

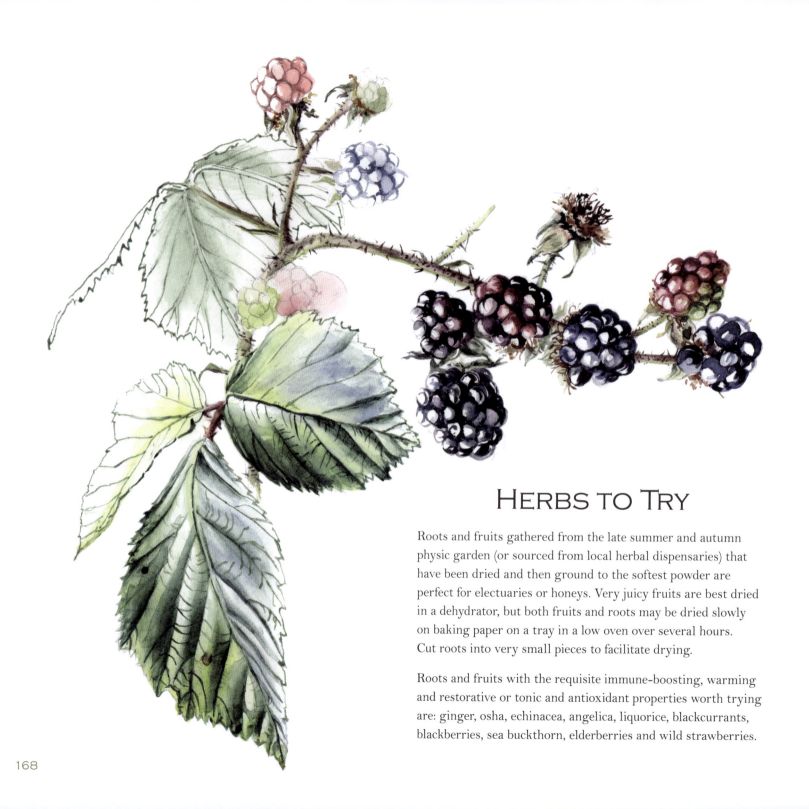

HERBS TO TRY

Roots and fruits gathered from the late summer and autumn physic garden (or sourced from local herbal dispensaries) that have been dried and then ground to the softest powder are perfect for electuaries or honeys. Very juicy fruits are best dried in a dehydrator, but both fruits and roots may be dried slowly on baking paper on a tray in a low oven over several hours. Cut roots into very small pieces to facilitate drying.

Roots and fruits with the requisite immune-boosting, warming and restorative or tonic and antioxidant properties worth trying are: ginger, osha, echinacea, angelica, liquorice, blackcurrants, blackberries, sea buckthorn, elderberries and wild strawberries.

A Simple Electuary Recipe

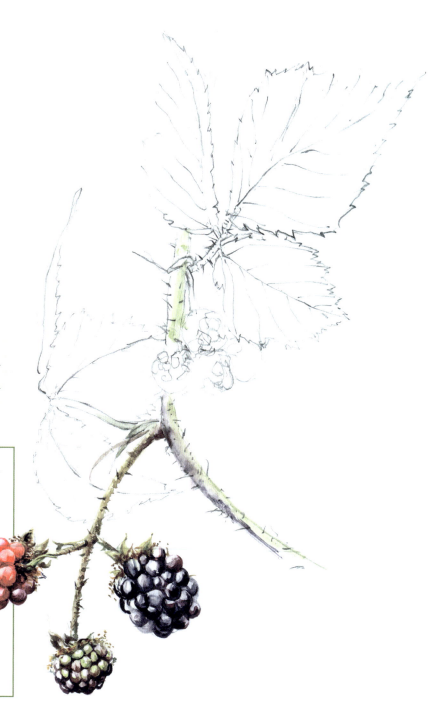

Ingredients

2 tsp dried powdered herb(s) – see suggestions opposite

Enough honey to fill the jar

How to Make

- Place dried powdered herb(s) into a clean, empty honey jar
- Pour in sufficient honey to fill the remainder of the jar
- Date, lid and label

How to Take

One teaspoon as required – up to three times a day.

Storage

The honey will thicken with time and should store well.

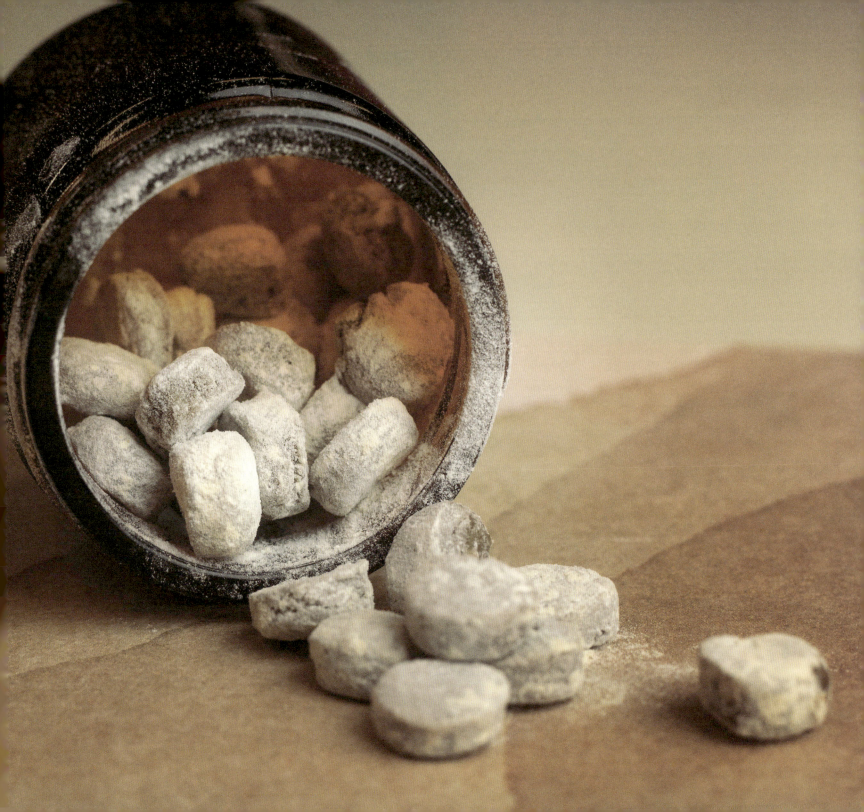

VII.
LOZENGES &
COUGH MIXTURES

LOZENGES

Lozenges (or 'troches' as they were originally known), resembling small medicinal cakes, are believed to have originated in ancient Egypt, where they are most likely to have been made from honey flavoured with lemon, botanicals and spices. Passing down through the classical world of the Greek physicians, such as Galen and the dispensaries of a thousand unknown apothecaries, they have remained little changed in all this time and are still being prepared by both our herbal and orthodox contemporary pharmacists.

We love lozenges for many reasons: first – the joy of which should never be underestimated – lozenges are simply such good fun to make! Second, they provide an exciting and quite rare opportunity for us to work a favourite piece of *Materia medica* – the gums!

Gums are extraordinarily lovely compounds to work. Their crystalline structure enables them to be crushed down into fine, glistening particles or various grades of softly ground powder, depending on the gums themselves and what is required of them.

Their readily water-soluble, highly demulcent and soothing nature makes them an easy as well as functional ingredient to incorporate into our lozenge-making practices. Therapeutically, they are widely appreciated as suspending, thickening, emulsifying and binding agents.

Gums are produced in different parts of botanicals through a process known as gummosis (the oozing of sap) that usually occurs as a healing response to some wound or other damage

(e.g. a canker) that has been sustained. Such gummy exudences are very common on fruit trees – especially those bearing stone fruits, such as cherry, sloe, plum, etc.

Gum arabic was the first gum to be introduced into the herbology remedy making taking place here at Royal Botanic Garden Edinburgh. Some of the finest we ever received reached us directly from the exuberant bazaars of the Arabian Peninsula, where munificent supplies were discovered and brought back by our former director of learning and horticulture, Leigh Morris. From that point onwards, a once very small glasshouse sapling of *Acacia senegal* (native to sub-Saharan Africa) – gnarly and thorny though it was, like so much of the flora of Arabia – became the object of our enduring affection.

But back to lozenges… we have a practical need for them, yet for so many years a truly successful lozenge recipe illuded us. We lost ourselves in the medicinal apothecary-styled candies, comfits and confections of the past until a traditional 17th-century recipe by Elizabeth Jenner in *For Making of Waters and Syrups and Other Physical Remedies* (1706) suddenly came to light, whose ingredients, measures and method of preparation were almost exactly what we were after. Here is that recipe, adapted and reproduced by kind permission of Susan Rennie.

Tragacanth Gum Lozenges Recipe

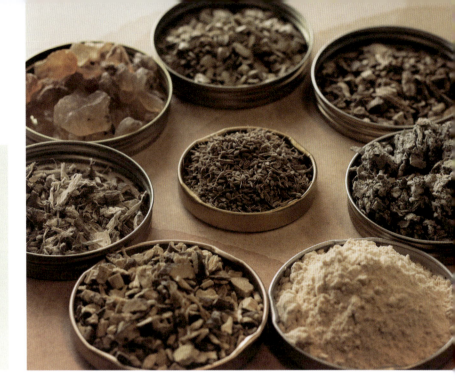

Ingredients

1 tbsp elecampane root

100ml rosewater (food safe)

225g golden (unrefined) icing sugar

½ tsp tragacanth gum powder

10g liquorice root powder

5g orris root powder

5g anise seeds

5g angelica (*Angelica archangelica*) seeds

How to Make

- Make an infusion by steeping the elecampane root in rosewater overnight, then strain and reserve the liquid

- Sift the icing sugar into a bowl and add the powdered tragacanth, liquorice and orris

- Crush the anise and angelica seeds in a pestle and mortar and add to the powdered mixture

- Add enough of the rosewater infusion to form a stiff paste

- Dust a flat surface with icing sugar and roll out the mixture to a thickness of around 5mm

- Cut out rounds using a small cutter (or use a tailor's thimble for historical authenticity!)

- Place the lozenges on a plate or baking tray to dry

- When they have hardened, dust them liberally with icing sugar

How to Take

One lozenge orally, as needed. Allow to dissolve slowly.

Storage

Store in a lidded tin or jar.

Author's note: *These lozenges are not only (deliciously!) comforting for the sore throat, they are also effective as a cough remedy. The main aromatic powdered root ingredients of liquorice, elecampane and orris have among them demulcent, anti-inflammatory, antiviral, antiseptic, antitussive (effective against a tickly cough) and expectorant properties, which are perfectly complemented by the soothing, pleasant flavour of the rosewater. We hope you will enjoy them as much as we do!*

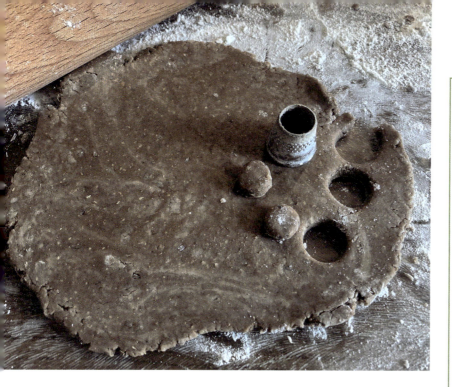

COLTSFOOT COUGH DROPS RECIPE

As not everyone likes liquorice and aniseed flavours, we made a version that uses finely powdered coltsfoot (*Tussilago farfara*, a traditional cough sweet ingredient), which proved equally good…

INGREDIENTS

2 tbsp elecampane root
40ml rosewater (infused with elecampane root pieces)
1 tbsp dried coltsfoot herb and flowers
125g icing sugar
½ tsp tragacanth gum powder
1 tsp orris root powder
1 tsp angelica seeds
Slippery elm powder (to thicken the mixture)

HOW TO MAKE

- Infuse the elecampane root in rosewater overnight
- In the morning, strain out the root
- Grind the coltsfoot to a very fine, soft powder
- Sift the icing sugar, tragacanth, orris and coltsfoot into a bowl
- Add the finely ground, sifted angelica seeds to the other powdered ingredients
- Stir to combine the ingredients
- Add the rosewater and mix the ingredients carefully together
- Add sufficient slippery elm powder to thicken the mixture into a dough
- Dust icing sugar evenly onto a flat surface
- Roll out the mixture to a 5mm thickness
- Using a tailor's thimble, cut out the lozenges
- Place on a plate or tray, dusted liberally with icing sugar, and allow to dry
- When hardened, dust with more icing sugar

HOW TO TAKE

One lozenge orally, as needed. Allow to dissolve slowly.

STORAGE

Store in a lidded tin or jar.

Author's note: *Coltsfoot rock may still be found in some old-fashioned sweet shops, but it is no longer made using real coltsfoot – it has become just a hard-boiled sweet flavoured with, rather ironically, aniseed!*

TROCHES OF VIPERS

A recipe found in the 1721 edition of the *London Pharmacopoeia* for 'white pectoral lozenges' is so fundamentally close to our own (see p. 172) in its key ingredients that it reveals the perpetuity of particular elements of our *Materia medica*, past and present. One cannot help but wonder how far-reaching the influence of the then-orthodox *Medicine Maker's Handbook* has become. Then we come upon a host of other lozenge recipes with ingredients that seem far more typical of the time, with one that definitely captures the (non-vegan) imagination! Below are the instructions for a 'Troches of Vipers':

> Take half a pound of Viper's flesh, separated from the skins, the entrails, the fat, the heads and the tails, and boiled till it grows soft in Spring-water, seasoned with a little Dill and Salt, and afterwards clear'd of the backbone; of bisket Bread, ground and searced, two ounces; beat them up together, with a proper quantity of the broth, remaining after the vipers were boiled, into a mass, to be formed into Troches, according to art.

I love the use of spring water here (which seems so contemporary and unexpected) and the light seasoning of dill and salt, which is almost humorous given the context!

A footnote follows the recipe in the 1721 edition of the *Pharmacopoeia*: 'These Troches are brought to us from other parts, ready prepared; but the dried flesh of the viper is with justice preferred thereto.'

Don't try this at home!

COUGH MIXTURES

Similar to our quest for the perfect lozenge, the formulation of a herbology cough mixture that was both effective as a medicine and equally good to take off the spoon became something of a *cause célèbre*. Many of our favourite old herbals were revisited and innumerable combinations of 'the cough mixture herbs' (pp. 176–177) were eagerly decocted into various bubbling pots of thick honeys, treacles and syrups, only to be sampled, disclaimed over (like the one that was effectively a 'syrup of turnips'!) and discarded. Some in truth came close to what we were after but none absolutely nailed it, until this one. It has become known as 'Catherine's Croupy Cough Mixture' – nothing at all to do with myself but the fine work of another herbologist, Catherine Sanderson, to whom we are eternally grateful for this recipe – now a staple in our herbology autumn/winter green pharmacy and with only a very few tiny (but essential) tweaks.

Despite what Bartram (1998) notes, the traditional English cough syrup mixture 'holy trinity' of horehound, hyssop and honey can be extremely bitter due to the horehound (*Marrubium vulgare*), an incredibly difficult ingredient to work with – arguably the most unpleasant of bitters, we have learnt the hard way how to handle it – i.e., as sparingly as possible!

We love the seeming complexity (and delicious synergy) that this recipe affords with regard to its expansive use of the cough remedy herbs and other desirable *Materia medica*. In a most satisfying way, it enables the medicine maker to sample and work with a complementary variety of ingredients all at once, and to elicit their best possible effects into one final mixture.

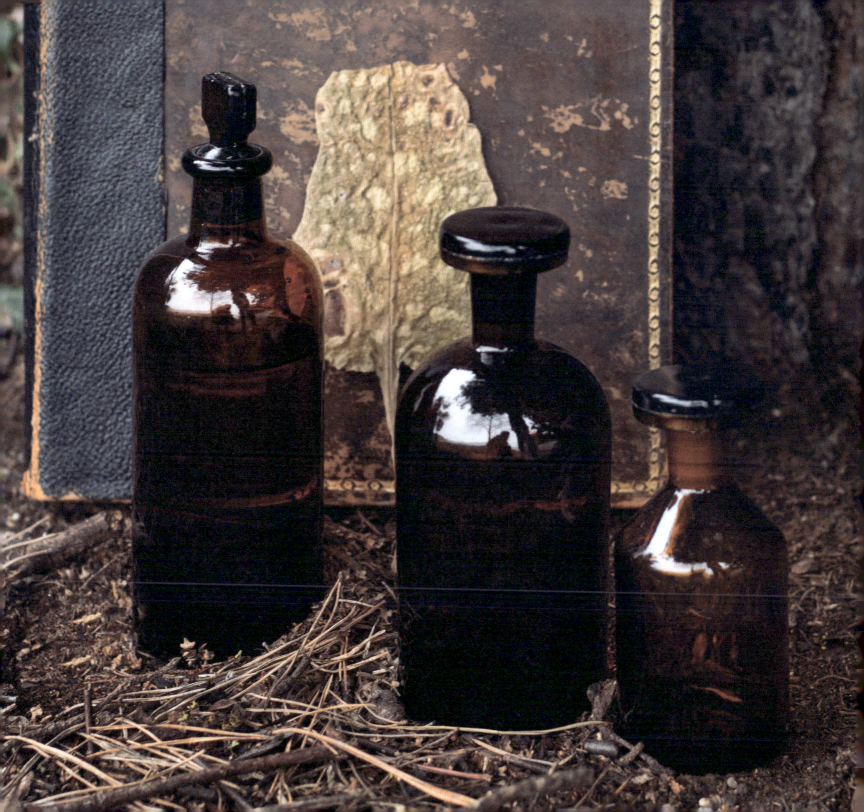

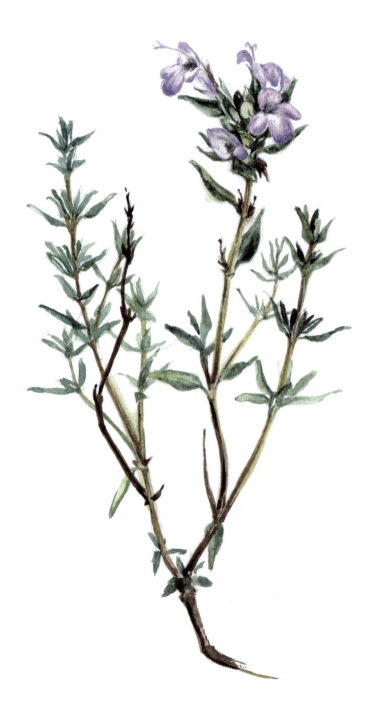

Cough Mixture Herbs

Here are some of the cough mixture herbs we most frequently reference as part of our herbology programme:

Aniseed (*Pimpinella anisum*)
The distinctively flavoured seeds of anise are a traditional ingredient in cough remedy formulations, where their accumulative effects are gently expectorant.

Balm of gilead buds (*Populus* x *gileadensis*)
Alcoholic extracts of the beautifully fragrant and resinous poplar buds are used to make an expectorant cough remedy that is usually prepared as a simple (on its own).

Coltsfoot (*Tussilago farfara*)
A classic cough remedy ingredient; the soft dried leaf and flower are used to add a relaxing, demulcent and expectorant note to any mixture.

Elecampane (*Inula helenium*)
The exquisitely aromatic inula root is used in cough mixtures as a warming and stimulating expectorant to ease the bronchial congestion of old coughs.

Horehound (*Marrubium vulgare*)
The bitter one! The flowering tops and leaf of white horehound (not black horehound) are something of a classic cough mixture (chest remedy) ingredient.

Hyssop (*Hyssopus officinalis*)
An excellent and gentle expectorant for children, this attractive purple-blue flowered herb holds mucilage, volatile oils and resins. It is good for all sorts of bronchial troubles.

ICELAND MOSS (*Cetraria islandica*)
Not a moss at all but a fascinating lichen that has the potential
to be a very soothing, demulcent and antitussive ingredient in a
cough mixture remedy.

LIQUORICE ROOT (*Glycyrrhiza glabra*)
A sweet and warming demulcent, liquorice is a soothing
expectorant and is distinctively flavoursome.

MARSHMALLOW ROOT (*Althaea officinalis*)
Marshmallow root is one of the most soothing and demulcent
of the antitussives. One of our favourites.

MULLEIN (*Verbascum thapsus*)
This statuesque botanical has the softest, downiest leaf and
a stunning yellow flower spike, both of which may be used to
make herbal cough mixtures.

PLEURISY ROOT (*Asclepias tuberosa*)
A beautiful physic garden botanical and a fantastic remedy for
the more tediously persistent and chronic cough that just won't
go away.

THYME (*Thymus vulgaris*)
The antiseptic dried leaf and flowering tops of common thyme
make this a valuable ingredient in any expectorant cough
mixture where there is underlying infection.

WILD CHERRY BARK (*Prunus serotina*)
An antitussive, generally prepared as a simple for tickly coughs
and a favourite remedy for children, as it does indeed taste
of cherries!

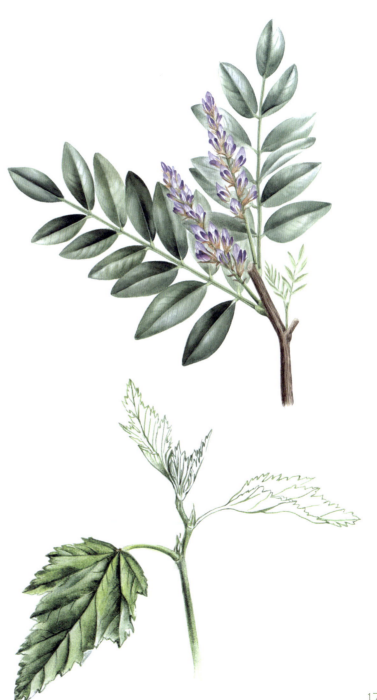

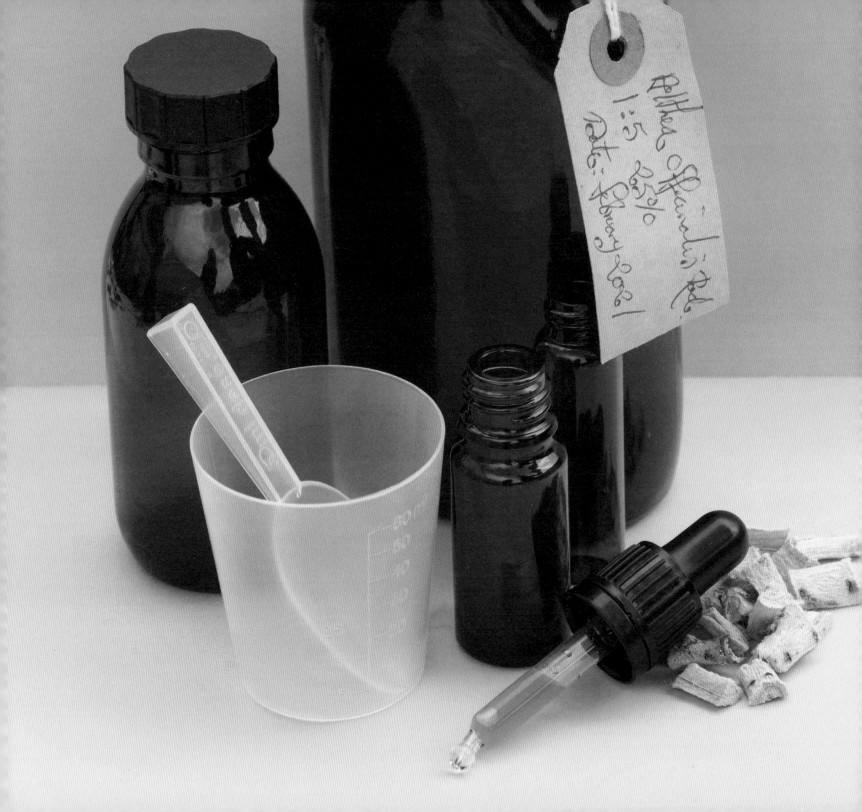

Althea officinalis Rt.
1:5 25%
note: february 2021

CATHERINE'S CROUPY COUGH MIXTURE RECIPE

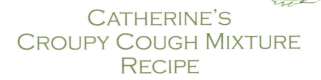

INGREDIENTS
(FOR THE BASE MIXTURE)

20g dried liquorice root pieces

20g dried marshmallow root pieces

900ml cold water

500g raw cane sugar

1 tbsp molasses

1 tbsp honey

Optional: 2 tbsp ginger root syrup,
12 drops of liquorice root fluid extract, or peel of
1 mandarin or a bitter Seville orange

COUGH MIXTURE HERBS
Choose your own from the following:

5g dried anise

5g dried hyssop

3g dried thyme

3g dried mullein

3g dried coltsfoot

½g dried horehound
(just a token gesture or ignore altogether – it's ever so bitter!)

HOW TO MAKE

- Grind the liquorice and marshmallow root pieces in a pestle and mortar
- Place in a pan
- Add 900ml cold water and stir
- Allow to stand for one hour
- Add the dried herb ingredients of your choice
- Simmer the mixture until reduced by half
- Strain out the herbs and measure the remaining liquid
- Return this decoction to the pan
- Add the sugar, molasses and ginger root syrup
- Simmer over gentle heat until sugar dissolves
- Stir in the honey
- Remove from the heat
- Add the liquorice root fluid extract
- Mix well using a wooden spoon
- Pour into sterilised syrup jars, lid and label

HOW TO TAKE

One teaspoon as needed, up to five times a day.

STORAGE

Store in a refrigerator and use within a fortnight.

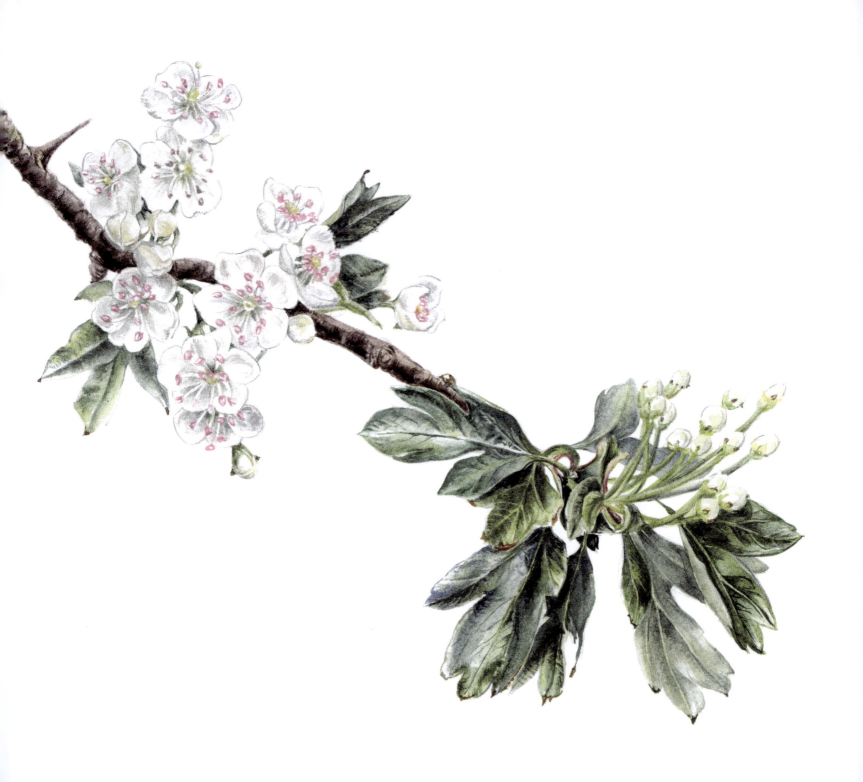

VIII.
HERBAL CONFECTIONARIES & COMFITS

FRUIT LEATHERS

Although it might at first seem that fruit leather is not the sort of thing that would appear in a 17th-century herbal or pharmacopoeia, dried fruit goods may be traced far back in antiquity to the ancient Persian and later Arabic culinary arts.

Fruit leathers may be made from all sorts of delicious fruits, including many of the wild hedgerow berries such as elderberry, sea buckthorn, blackberry and rosehip (with all those hairy little seeds removed!). If gathering berries from the wild, always ensure that a plentiful supply remains for little creatures and birds, substituting some of the wild berries for alternative, more readily sourced and abundant fruits. Indeed, some of the very best recipes may be compounded from a medley of fruit pulps made up from any of the following: apricots, plums, apples, pears, blackcurrants, blaeberries, damsons, sloes, raspberries, strawberries, peaches, grapes – even rhubarb!

It's easy to get carried away by all the exciting (not to mention colourful) possibilities, and there are lots of alternative recipes out there. Just remember that at least some of the more pectin-rich fruits are required to ensure that the pulp sets – crab apples, unripe blackberries and hawthorn berries are all good for this purpose. Sugar is not an essential ingredient for most contemporary fruit leathers, unless the fruits or berries used are particularly sour.

Our fruit leather recipe references one of the most magical (sacred) trees of our *Materia medica*: the hawthorn. Recognised as one of nature's most restorative heart tonics, it has been found to nurture normal heart function. The heart is so much more than just a physiological pump, though; it has another often-forgotten role as an organ of perception. This is something the ancient Egyptians and other cultures seem to have been intuitively aware of; hence perhaps the origins of our own concepts of the 'broken heart'.

There are many delightful hawthorn remedies that can be taken to comfort the heart, whose profoundly recuperative effects may be greatly complemented by the soothing, cooling and anti-inflammatory properties of either a marshmallow root or rose petal extract. To this end, our hawthorn fruit leather formula has proven to be one of our most endearing and deeply appreciated fruit-based remedies and confections.

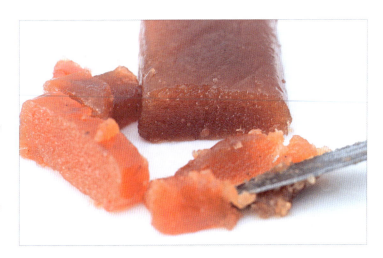

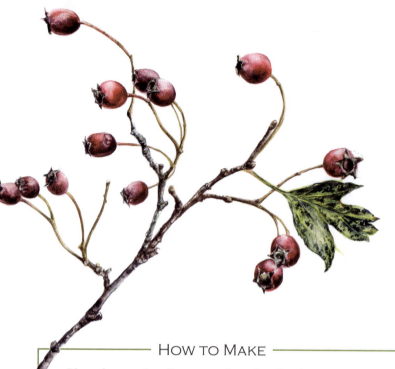

Hawthorn Fruit Leather Recipe

Ingredients

3 tbsp marshmallow root pieces

1 litre cold water
(this could be lightly infused with apothecary rose petals)

1 lime

475g fresh hawthorn berries

225g raw cane sugar

1 cinnamon stick

How to Make

- Place the marshmallow root pieces in a bowl and cover with cold water
- Allow to stand and infuse overnight
- Strain into a jug
- Warm the oven at its lowest setting
- Squeeze the lime and set the juice to one side
- Pour the marshmallow infusion into a pan
- Add the hawthorn berries, sugar and cinnamon stick
- Gently bring the ingredients to the boil
- Simmer gently for 20 minutes, or until soft
- Remove the cinnamon stick
- Blend in a liquidiser with the lime juice
- Strain the mixture through a sieve to remove any remaining haw pips (these should never be consumed)
- Pour into a greaseproof-paper-lined baking tray, to a thickness of about 1cm
- Allow to dry in the heated oven for several hours, ideally overnight or until chewy and leave to cool
- Cut into strips or roll into curls

How to Take

Suck or chew on a piece of fruit leather whenever you like – they are healthy, nutritious and totally yummy.

Storage

Wrap your fruit leather in greaseproof paper and store in an airtight box or tin.

Author's note: *If the recipe is made purely from hawthorn berries, as above (with no other fruits), do not consume more than around three (maximum five) 2.5cm pieces daily. The oligomeric procyanidin compounds (OPCs) that hawthorn holds have been shown to exert positively inotropic and negatively chronotropic effects upon the heart – this means that hawthorn has the capacity to slightly raise the heart rate, while it gently slows and regulates its rhythm. However, if taken in high doses, hawthorn may cause low blood pressure and sedation. Always consult a doctor before taking any botanicals known to exert an influence upon the heart and circulatory system.*

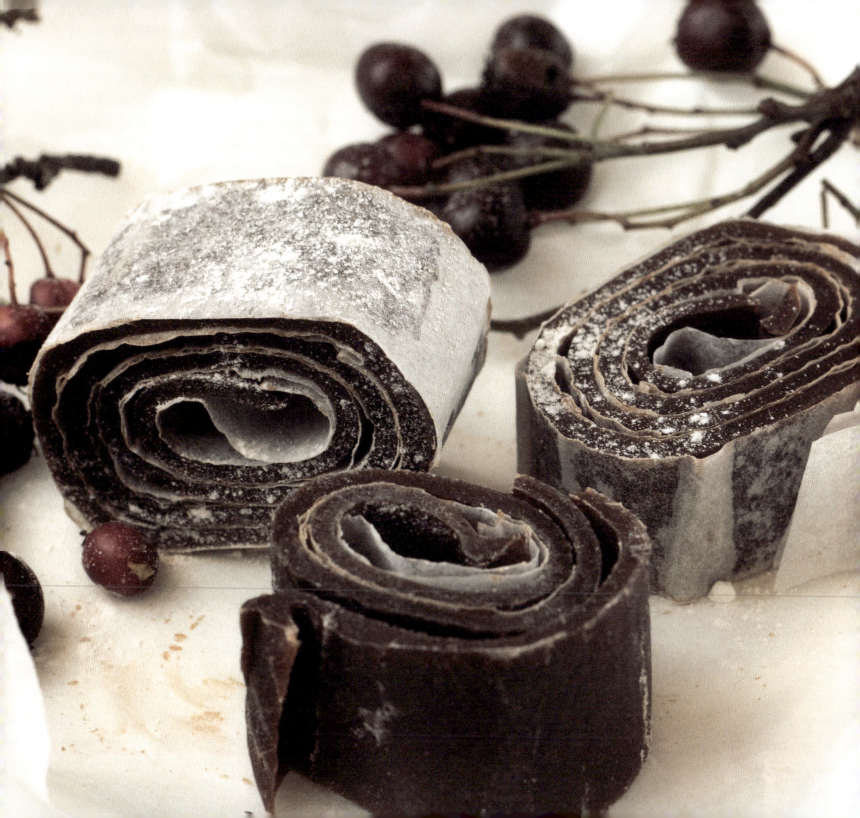

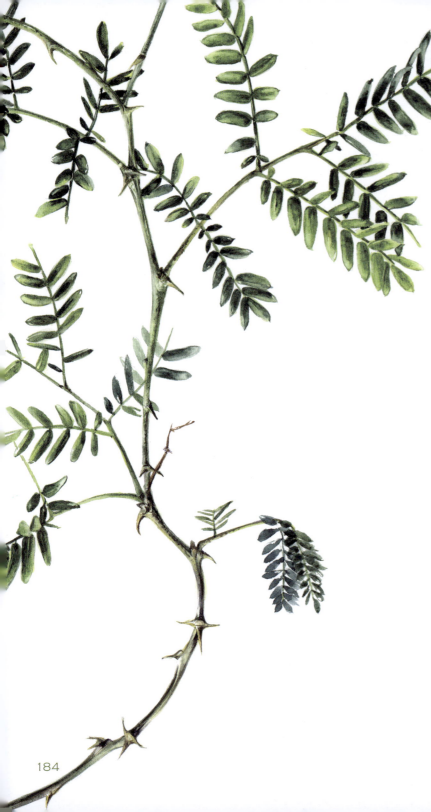

COMFITS

Comfits were (and are still) aromatic seeds (such a caraway, fennel or anise), nuts or small pieces of spice that have been coated in several hardened layers of a sugar syrup solution. They are one of the earliest forms of sugar confectionary and first began to appear during the medieval period, as highly sought, sweet and flavoursome remedies for indigestion.

Comfits could be either smooth (pearl or plain round) or ragged in appearance, depending on how they were made. Ragged comfits were created when the sugar was 'of a high decoction', i.e. very hot and poured from a greater height, which gave a rougher texture.

Comfits made from caraway seeds seem to have been the most popular in England. These were enjoyed as a comforting (how appropriate!) digestive remedy, probably with some spiced wine as a postprandial, when their warming carminative effects would help to prevent indigestion and wind.

Please note that comfits are quite time-consuming to make, but are so worth the effort if you can be bothered! The following is a favourite recipe.

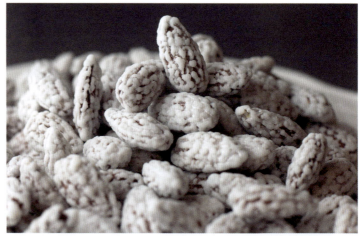

TWELFTH NIGHT COMFITS RECIPE

Whichever ingredient you choose – whether aromatic seeds, strips of citrus peel or particles of spices – it is recommended (but not essential) that you incorporate some gum arabic (dissolved in rosewater). This will help the sugar syrup adhere more readily – especially if you are making cinnamon comfits. We have included instructions for How to Make this solution first.

INGREDIENTS

1 tsp gum arabic powder (or gum tragacanth powder)

3 tsp rosewater

1 tbsp aromatic seeds (e.g. caraway, aniseed, fennel)

200g sugar (raw cane or white sugar)

80ml cold water

HOW TO MAKE

- Allow the gum to dissolve in the rosewater overnight, yielding a thick, gummy solution

  If you do choose to coat your ingredients with gum arabic, do this in the first few charges (coats) of syrup – use six parts sugar syrup to one part gum arabic solution

- Warm the seeds in a big flat-bottomed pan (like a griddle)

- Heat the sugar and water in a separate pan, until the sugar has completely dissolved

- Gather the seeds together into a small heap in the middle of the pan using a wooden spoon

- Take 1 tsp of sugar solution and pour it over the seeds – this may not seem much, but be patient

- Using the back of the wooden spoon, stir the seeds until the sugar dries (if you use too much syrup, the seeds will stick together – less is more!)

- After the first few charges of syrup, the seeds will gradually begin to turn white

- After about ten charges, you are done – don't attempt to add more syrup than this

- Allow the comfits to dry properly overnight (at least eight hours)

- At this point, you will have already made a myriad of tiny comfits and you could stop here. However, you can make more sugar syrup solution and coat your seeds again and again!

- The bigger the comfits get, the more you will need to divide your batch – you need to be able to work comfortably with the pan

HOW TO TAKE

Consume as needed to ease dyspepsia, or just enjoy as an aromatic sweet and invigorating breath freshener.

STORAGE

Once the comfits are ready and you are happy with them, store in small lidded tins or jars. Comfits made in this way will keep for several years.

CINNAMON COMFITS RECIPE

INGREDIENTS

2–3 Ceylon cinnamon sticks

Gum arabic solution
(see Twelfth Night Comfits Recipe, p. 185)

200g raw cane or white sugar

80ml cold water

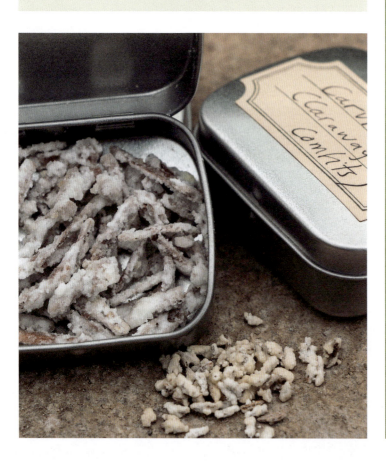

HOW TO MAKE

- Infuse the cinnamon sticks overnight in water to soften

- Cut the cinnamon into the thinnest needle-like strips

- Allow the cinnamon to dry thoroughly and completely

- Coat the cinnamon with the gum arabic or syrup solution in the first three charges

- Allow the comfits to dry properly (overnight) after about eight charges of syrup

- Make another solution of sugar syrup the following morning, and proceed as in the Twelfth Night Comfits Recipe

HOW TO TAKE

Consume as needed to ease dyspepsia, or take as a sweet, invigorating aromatic breath freshener.

STORAGE

Once the comfits are ready and you are happy with them, store in small lidded tins or jars. These comfits will keep for several years.

Author's note: *Sugared almonds are a familiar form of comfit that are still very much with us. Rather confusingly, these used to be referred to as 'sugared plums' – a name that was given to any of the bigger comfits and therefore frequently nothing at all to do with preserved plum fruits that are candied and crystalised with sugar – as lovely as they sound!*

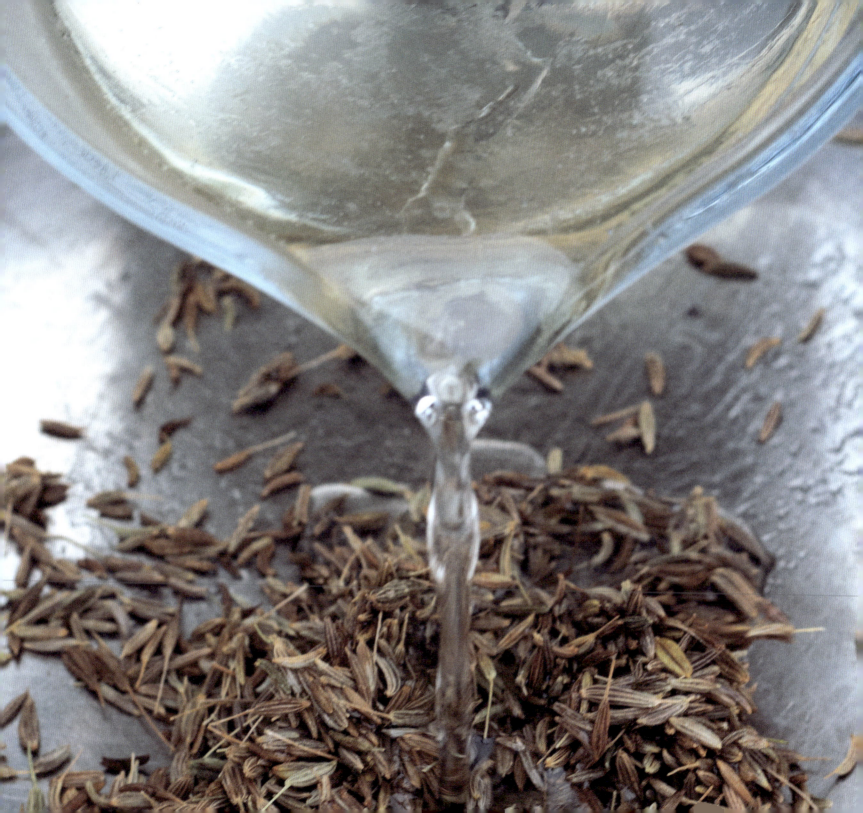

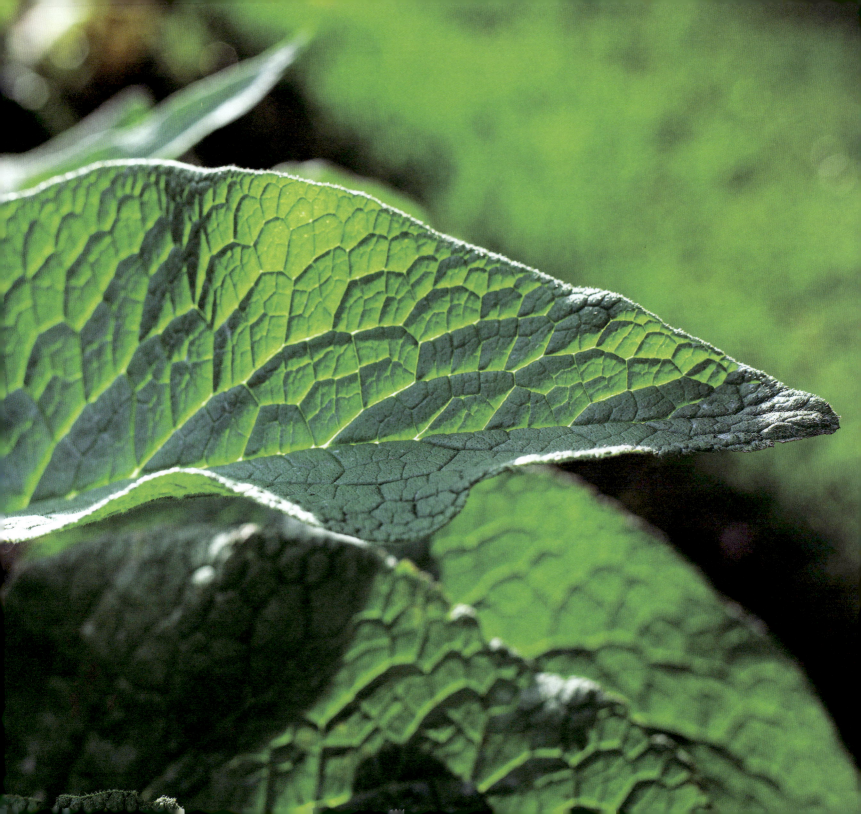

IX.

COMFREY ROOT BALM

Every year, just before the earth becomes too cold and frozen by the first hoar frosts, we bundle up and head out into the Garden to dig up some comfrey root. It has become something of a ritual, which, however inclement the darkening afternoon, we all seem to enjoy – not least because the root itself, like most other roots of substance (and even some of the more spindly ones), can be a really satisfying pleasure to exhume, affording a particularly memorable preliminary remedy making moment.

Comfrey (*Symphytum officinale*) seems to have always been with us. The great-great-great-grandfather of all vulneraries, it must surely be one of our best loved and most resoundingly effective of all wound healers. Sutherland naturally had comfrey in his 17th-century medicinal physic garden and it is unsurprisingly no stranger in the *Materia medica* of the physician's pharmacopoeia of that time either.

Comfrey is arguably most renowned for its remarkable capacity to heal the body's connective tissues – from slow-to-heal wounds of the integumentary system to fractured or even broken bones. Several of its former common names (e.g. 'boneset') reflect its efficacy there. Allantoin, one of the most abundant compounds found in comfrey, is now recognised as being the most significant in augmenting its quite extraordinary healing effects, enhanced in no small part by a very tangible mucilage presence – the highly slippery nature of which makes the cutting of its freshly scrubbed roots quite perilous!

Here follows our recipe for the beautiful soft, white comfrey root balm that we make each autumn, temporarily disturbing the agency worms as we delve deep into the dark and digesting earth for our roots. As the light fades, grubby roots in hand, we return to the welcome warmth of the herbology room to begin our medicine making.

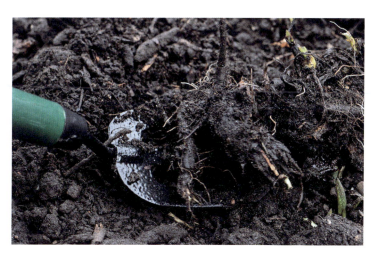

COMFREY ROOT BALM
RECIPE

INGREDIENTS

1 tbsp comfrey root
(ideally freshly dug, scrubbed and cut into small pieces)

Almond (or other base) oil – sufficient to half fill a
honey/jam jar and to submerge the herb

5 tsp per 100ml oil beeswax

3–5 drops essential oil
(e.g. lavender, tea tree, frankincense or eucalyptus)

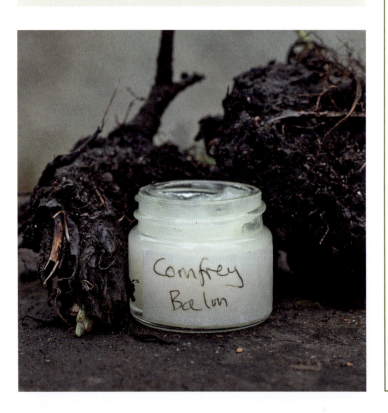

HOW TO MAKE

- Crush the comfrey root pieces and place in an empty honey/jam jar and cover with oil

- Stand the jar (with no lid) in a pan of warm water (creating a bain-marie), making sure the water only reaches about halfway up the jar

- Gently heat the water and allow to simmer for 20 minutes

- A metal utensil (e.g. a knife or long-handled spoon) placed in the jar will help prevent the balm from cracking

- Strain out the root and return the jar (with its now-infused oil) to the bain-marie

- Melt in the beeswax

- Carefully remove the jar from the pan, and allow the mixture to cool and solidify

- Once the ointment has formed, lid the jar and label

HOW TO USE

Apply topically, as needed, to help heal minor (cleansed) cuts and grazes, bruises and inflamed or generally irritated cutaneous tissues.

STORAGE

An ointment made to this simple herb, oil and wax formula should keep for several years, but all herbal remedies are best enjoyed when freshly made.

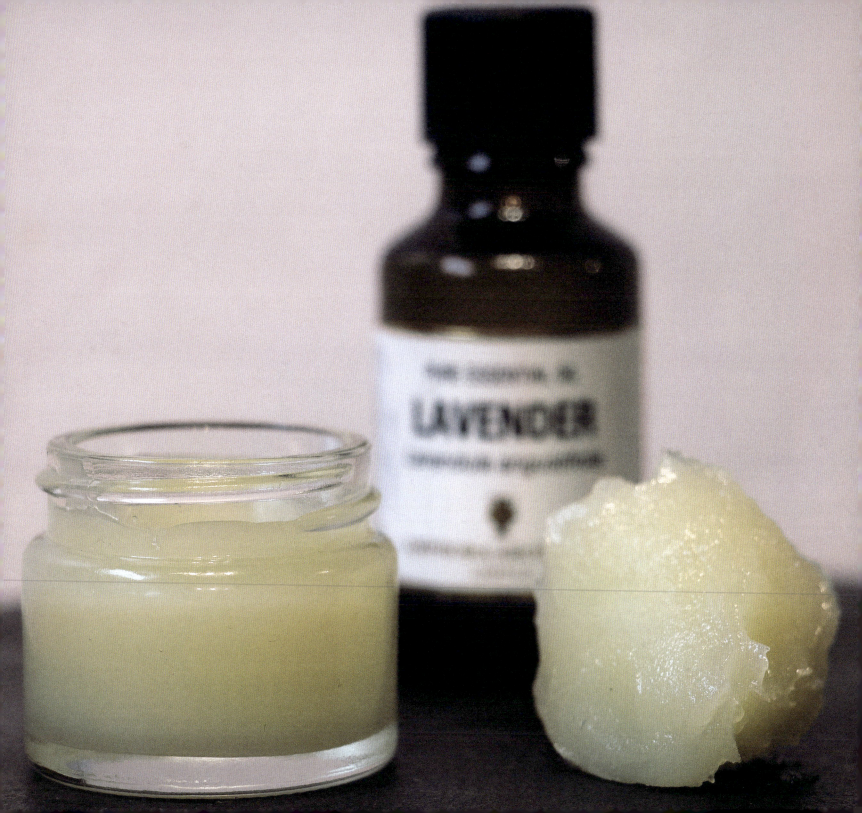

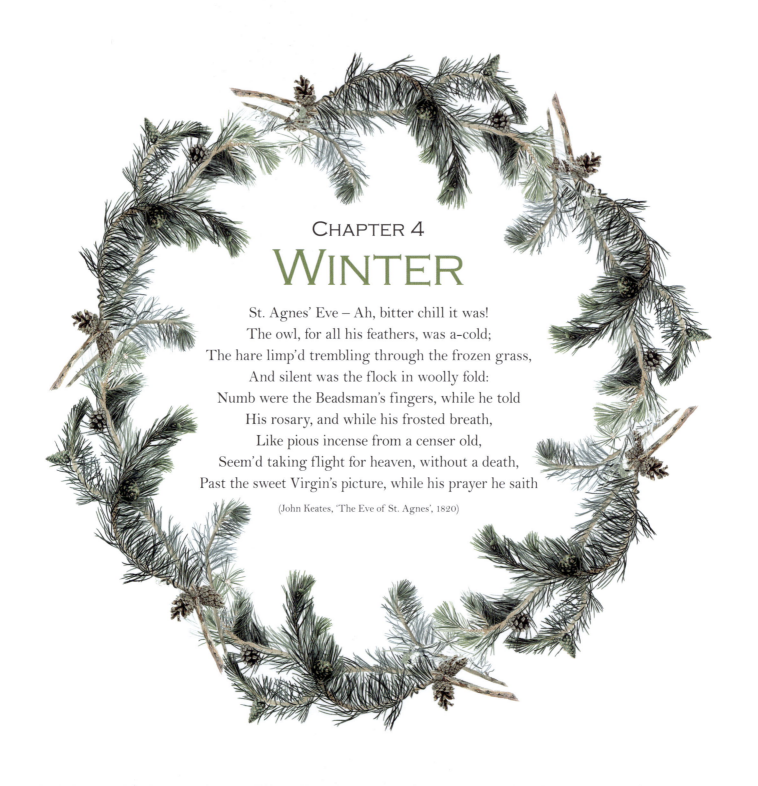

CHAPTER 4
WINTER

St. Agnes' Eve – Ah, bitter chill it was!
The owl, for all his feathers, was a-cold;
The hare limp'd trembling through the frozen grass,
And silent was the flock in woolly fold:
Numb were the Beadsman's fingers, while he told
His rosary, and while his frosted breath,
Like pious incense from a censer old,
Seem'd taking flight for heaven, without a death,
Past the sweet Virgin's picture, while his prayer he saith

(John Keates, 'The Eve of St. Agnes', 1820)

So, finally, it is winter and the earth sleeps. It seems as though all of nature's deepest rhythms have slowed as we enter the coldest, darkest moments of the year.

In the herbology physic garden, the tools have been put away in their storage trunk and the shed (with its happily undisturbed spiders in sleepy repose) is bolted until such times as it is needed again.

A quiet stillness descends over the grounds that were once so busy with the activity, camaraderie and chatter of bygone gardening.

Only our companionable little robin seems to hold custodianship now; faithful friend that he is, and one of many red-breasted guardians of the winter garden. He flits busily about, this way and that, finding his perch among the neighbouring apple and fruit trees, rather than on our wheelbarrow and fork handles of warmer times.

Our other much-loved Royal Botanic Garden Edinburgh familiar, Marley the cat, is rather more conspicuously absent. Only the tell-tale paw prints along the frosted paths that lead to his favourite glasshouse reveal his otherwise undisclosed whereabouts.

The hours of daylight have shortened and by late afternoon, the winter sun is already sinking low. A crimson orb of breathtaking beauty, it blushes the Western hemisphere with vivid fiery pink before it sinks rapidly from sight, abandoning the yet blazing heavens to leave only a trail of clouds that are laced with gold and the palest of turquoise twilights in its wake. Then, as the cool air of dusk descends, the first and brightest glittering star of the early evening appears, set close beside the ghostly white of a crescent moon.

Gazing upon it, and with the blessings of home, comfort and warmth to return to, it feels good to be alive – the spirit tingles and the earth turns. In the bitter cold, the ground is frozen beneath glistening frosts and – if the winter is all that it should be – glinting drifts of snow.

The winter winds begin to blow, soughing around as they do through the deepest and darkest of nights, roaring down chimneys and whistling around dwellings, as if to find a way in.

But before we know it, evergreens are everywhere and the end of the year with all of its Yuletide festivities, merry-making and gift-giving is upon us. 'Tis the season of goodwill and the time when even the smallest acts of kindness can mean so much; not just among ourselves but in the wider natural world we may be able to offer a little additional succour to the wildlife visiting our gardens during these shivering times. One of the easiest, most rewarding things to do is simply to remember to feed the birds.

So, yes, it is winter and the earth sleeps. The Garden at night lies silent in the moonlight, the bare branches of the silhouetted trees are shadowed across its lawns and cast ephemeral lattice works along deserted paths, among which only those nocturnal creatures who are not hibernating stir and hunt.

From up among the avenues of the Garden's pines, an owl hoots softly as a small, dark shape pads silently round the corner of the front range glasshouse and disappears into the darkness.

PHYSIC GARDEN DIARY

THINGS TO DO IN THE PHYSIC GARDEN

During the depths of winter, our herbology physic garden herb beds lie almost undisturbed. Only our little blue shed might on occasion be unlocked and revisited to retrieve the twine, canes or fleece needed to attend a wind-ravaged climber or an overchilled fellow.

There's something rather lovely about simply pottering around inside a shed – even a relatively small one – and appreciating how tidy and organised you left it the last time you were in there. Packets of seeds are sorted and proudly arranged before being put away again, with all the self-same satisfaction and care of the most avid of collectors. The empty crates used to dry all our tea botanicals of the summer are neatly stacked and waiting for such times as they might be filled with flowers again, while the gleam of polished tools for us remains unseen, until the lid is lifted on our storage trunk come spring.

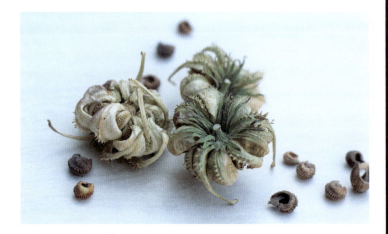

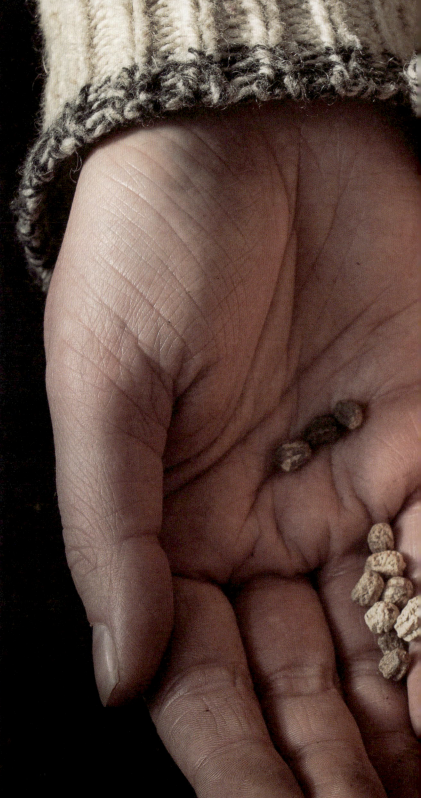

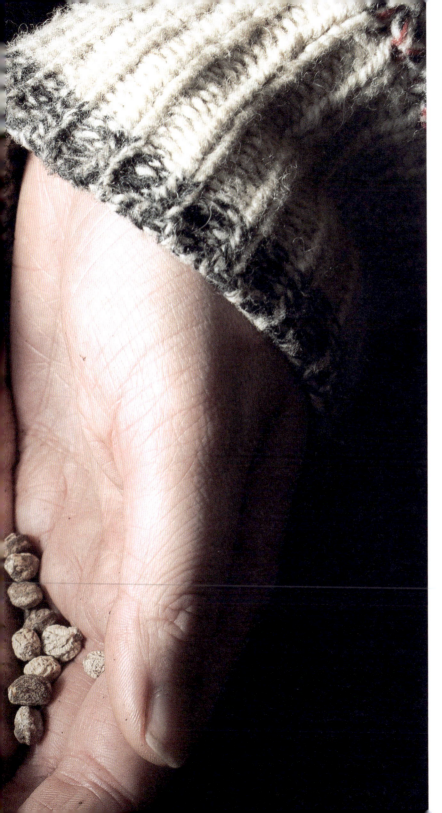

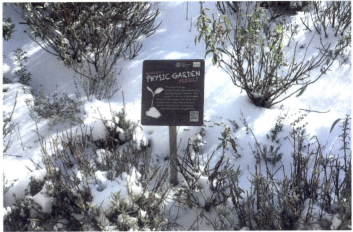

Here are some of the final tasks that may be undertaken in the garden in December, based on Evelyn's directions:

I.   'Continue to Trench Ground, and dung it', says Evelyn, to prepare the soil for the planting of fruit trees

II.   He advises: 'Either late in the month, or in January, prune, and cut all your Vine-shoots to the very root, save one, or two of the stoutest'

III.   'Turn and refresh your Autumnal Fruit, lest it taint, and open the windows where it lies, in clear and serene day'

IV.   Evelyn's final words for December and to conclude his *Kalendarium* are:

To impart both what we have experimentally learn'd by our own observations, and from others of undoubted Candor and Integrity: But of this, we promise a more ample Illustration, as it concerns the entire Art together with all its Ornaments of Use and magnificence, as these endeavors of ours shall find entertainment, and opportunity to contribute to the Design.

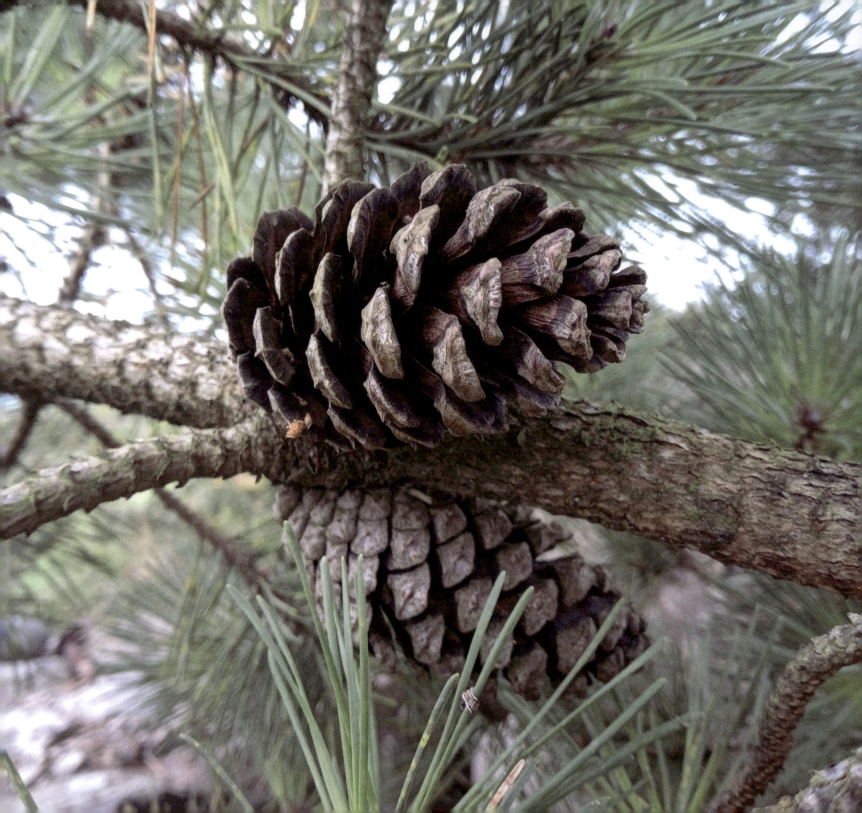

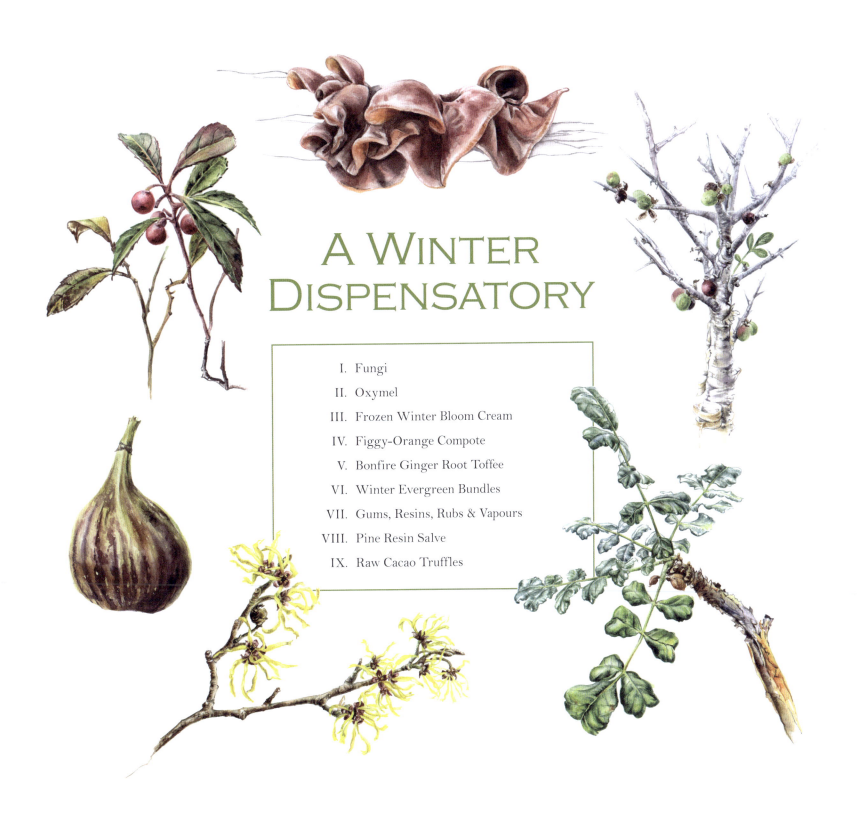

A WINTER DISPENSATORY

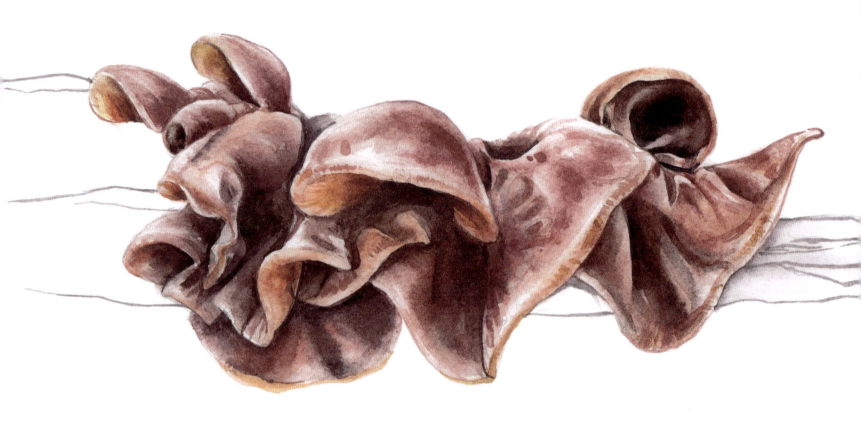

I.

FUNGI

At the Royal Botanic Garden Edinburgh, our herbology students are fortunate indeed to be introduced and encouraged to embrace the often quite literally magical *Materia medica* of medicinal mushrooms and fungi. What fascination do fungi hold for us? With their many ancient and folkloric associations (especially for those with psychotropic properties and distinctively appealing fruiting bodies, such as the *Amanita muscaria* and some of the *Psilocybe*), fungi belong to an extraordinary kingdom of organisms whose role in the sustenance of life, medicine and regeneration is finally acquiring the recognition it deserves.

The underground networks of mycelial communications between the trees in our woodlands and forests, which the fungi command, are enthralling. These delicate tangled 'webs' of natural transmission may be similarly found as friends, not foes, within the earth of our own gardens. Fungi in one form or another are, it seems, thankfully almost everywhere.

So, we simply had to have a fungi recipe in this book. How perfect that the very fungi we most wanted to feature is one of only two mentioned in the *Edinburgh Pharmacopoeia* (1699): 'jelly ears' (*Auricularia auricula-judae*). A contemporary liqueur chocolate concoction to warm the cochleae (sorry!) of the fungi connoisseur's heart, I would very much like to dedicate this recipe to Monica Wilde. But before we proceed any further, it must be said, be warned!

Jelly ear fungi really do resemble 'jelly ears', but don't let that put you off. This characterful little thing is definitely one of our fungi friends. Given its morphology and habit of growing almost exclusively on elder trees, it is easily distinguishable from the potentially more poisonous of the 'fungi foes' and it is, like most medicinal mushrooms, packed with beneficial compounds and potential therapeutic effects, not least for the function of the heart.

To name but a few, jelly ear fungi are exceptionally antioxidant, rich in B complex vitamins and immune-boosting polysaccharides. Their indigestible prebiotic fibres (in the form of ß-glucans) encourage the formation of those health-nurturing probiotics whose immensely supportive role in our digestive system (and wider metabolic) well-being is only now being fully appreciated.

The polysaccharides found in jelly ears (principally mannose, glucose, glucuronic acid and xylose) are known to inhibit platelet aggregation and blood clotting. While these can be highly desirable therapeutic effects, it is not recommended that you consume jelly ear fungi if you are already taking blood-thinning or anticoagulant medicines.

Author's note: *If gathering from the wild, it is imperative that you correctly identify the jelly ear, and only take sufficient for your needs – no more. Never gather from locations where there are only a few fungi in evidence. Remember to follow the forager's code of good practice.*

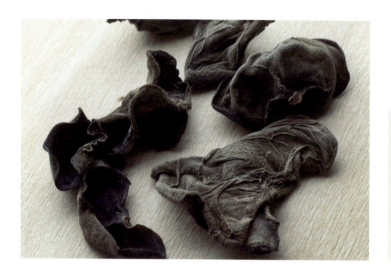

Chocolate Enfolded Auricles Recipe

Ingredients

1 handful fresh jelly ear fungi

Cherry or other fruit brandy liqueur of your choice
(to infuse the jelly ears)

Dark organic chocolate
(just enough to 'enfold' the jelly ears)

How to Make

- Rinse the jelly ears in cold water and gently blot dry with a soft tea towel
- Cover a cooling tray with a clean, soft tea towel and arrange the individual jelly ears to dry
- After two to three weeks, the jelly ears will have dehydrated sufficiently
- The jelly ears will shrink considerably during this time. Don't be alarmed; they will plump up again! (Jelly ears may be stored dried like this for up to a year)
- Next, steep the jelly ears in liqueur, until they are rehydrated and saturated with the liqueur. To do this, place the jelly ears in a bowl or zip-lock bag, ensuring they are fully immersed in the liqueur. (Note from Monica Wilde: if making these for children or recovering alcoholics, steep in orange juice)
- Leave the jelly ears to soak for around 12 hours, or until they have returned to their original volume – they should be plump and soft
- Once ready, shake gently to remove any drips of liqueur
- Blot dry very gently – take care not to squeeze out any of the liqueur

- Break the chocolate into small pieces and allow to melt slowly in a bain-marie
- Once the chocolate has melted, use a cocktail stick to dip your jelly ears
- Make sure you fully coat each fungi and twirl any excess chocolate off the back into the bowl
- Pin the cocktail sticks with their jelly ears into something like a florist's oasis block, covered in foil
- Allow to set

How to Take

Enjoy in moderation!

Storage

Store in an airtight container in the fridge and consume within a fortnight. They may be carefully removed from the cocktail sticks at this point.

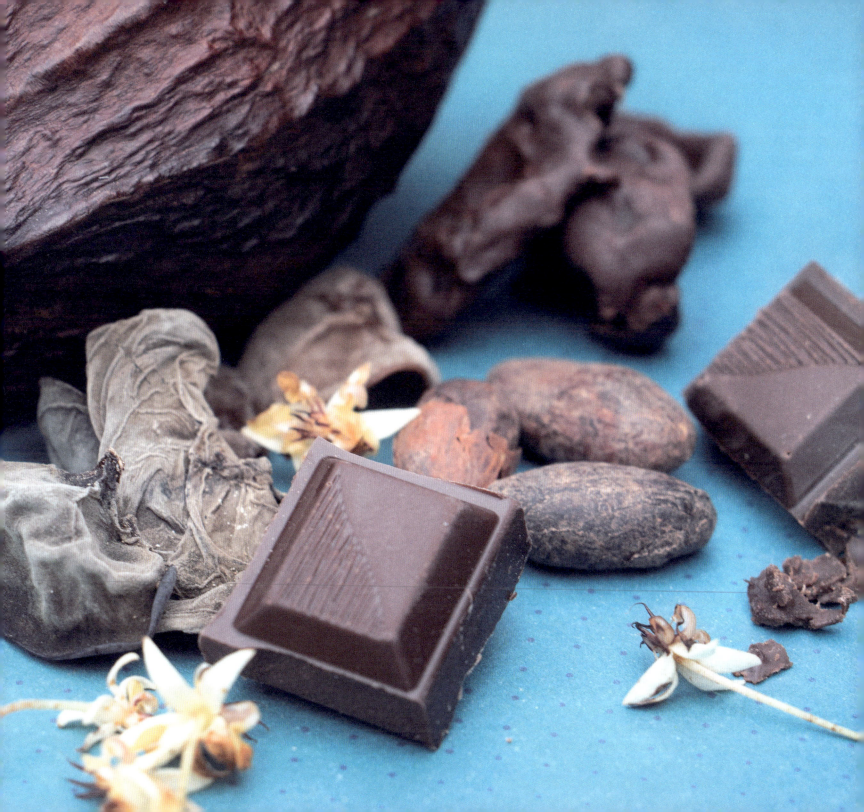

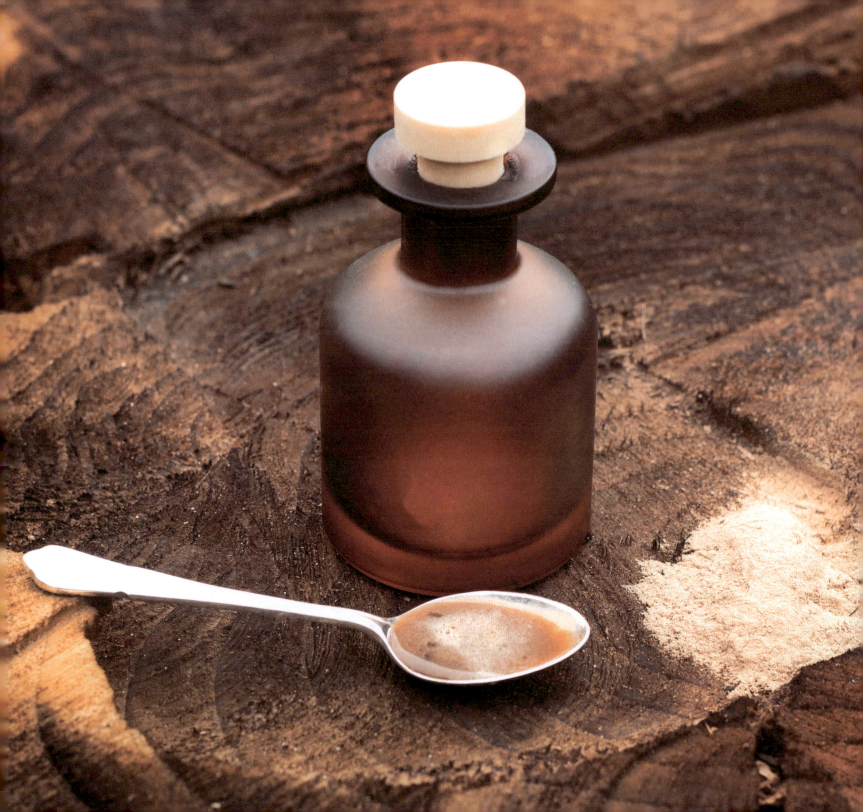

II.
OXYMEL

WHAT IS AN OXYMEL?

Oxymels are among some of the very oldest (and best) of our oral herbal remedies. They are believed to originate from ancient Persia and are made from a honey and vinegar base.

Recipes for oxymels abound throughout the 17th-century herbals, where the traditional meld of vinegar and honey is used simply on its own or with other medicinal ingredients decocted into it to make a delicious immune-boosting and restorative tonic remedy, perfect for winter.

A classic oxymel base is made from five parts honey to one part vinegar. The *Edinburgh Pharmacopoeia* (1699) includes an 'oxymel simplex' (simple oxymel) just after a rather lovely 'Honey of Roses' recipe, under the heading 'Mellita' (honeys).

Of all the *Materia medica* that we use throughout the herbology's green pharmacy remedy making, honey and apple cider vinegar are among the very best. Once melded together, their seismic therapeutic synergy is quite sufficient to make the simple oxymel base alone one of the most reinvigorating, remineralising and restorative herbal solutions known.

In the past, our herbology oxymels used to sometimes incorporate a dried medicinal arboreal ingredient, Pau d'Arco, to enhance the therapeutic effects of the overall mixture. This thousand-year-old Inca remedy became (and remains) a highly regarded immune booster, adaptogen and anticarcinogenic, extracted from the heartwood and inner bark of some trees native to South America.

Whenever such parts of a tree are sought after for medicine-making in the wild, it invariably spells disaster for those particular trees, and subsequently their indigenous forest habitat. A raised awareness of this, together with legitimate concerns surrounding the end quality of any *Materia medica* (product) that not only travels thousands of miles to reach us but which may not even have been properly identified or harvested and could be vulnerable to adulteration, prompts the need to carefully reconsider some of our ingredient choices. Please, be encouraged to do the same.

Pau d'Arco all too sadly exemplifies the trail of exploitation that can befall some of our most precious botanicals, and the unquantifiable collateral damage that so often ensues in its wake. Equally, learning about it can help to inform even the smallest, seemingly inconsequential decisions that we make, in a good way.

It is nearly always possible to find alternative, locally sourced and infinitely more sustainable botanicals with which to furnish our herbal remedies *and* it's fun to do so. As far as herbology goes, we have discontinued the use of Pau d'Arco for our oxymels in favour of roseroot (*Rhodiola rosea*), which now grows with a perpetually rewarding exuberance within the herbology herb beds of the Garden.

Here's our oxymel recipe that makes the most of roseroot's reputedly adaptogenic (fortifying tonic) effects compounded by the remineralising and nutritive effects of apple cider vinegar and organic honey.

Roseroot Oxymel
Recipe

Ingredients

100ml organic apple cider vinegar

20g dried roseroot (*Rhodiola rosea*),
astragalus or echinacea root

500g organic honey
(pure heather honey is highly recommended)

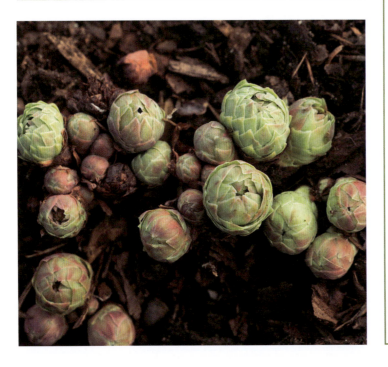

How to Make

- Put the vinegar and herb in a pot

- Simmer for 10 minutes

- Strain out the liquid and return to the pot

- Add the honey

- Warm gently until the mixture has the consistency of a syrup, stirring continuously throughout

- Once cool, pour into sterilised glass jars or bottles, lid and label

How to Take

Take a couple of teaspoons daily as a tonic.

Storage

An oxymel generally stores well, but it is recommended that you enjoy this remedy freshly made and consume within a fortnight.

Author's note: *Herbal ingredient measures will be variable depending on individual dosage recommendations and the nature of the medicinal plant being used.*

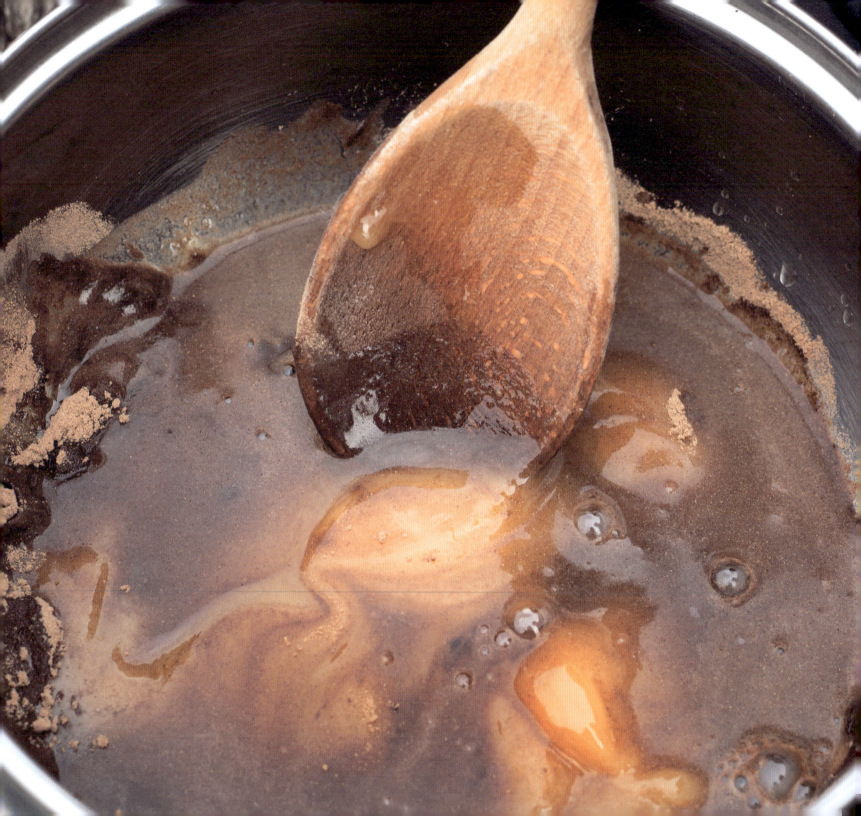

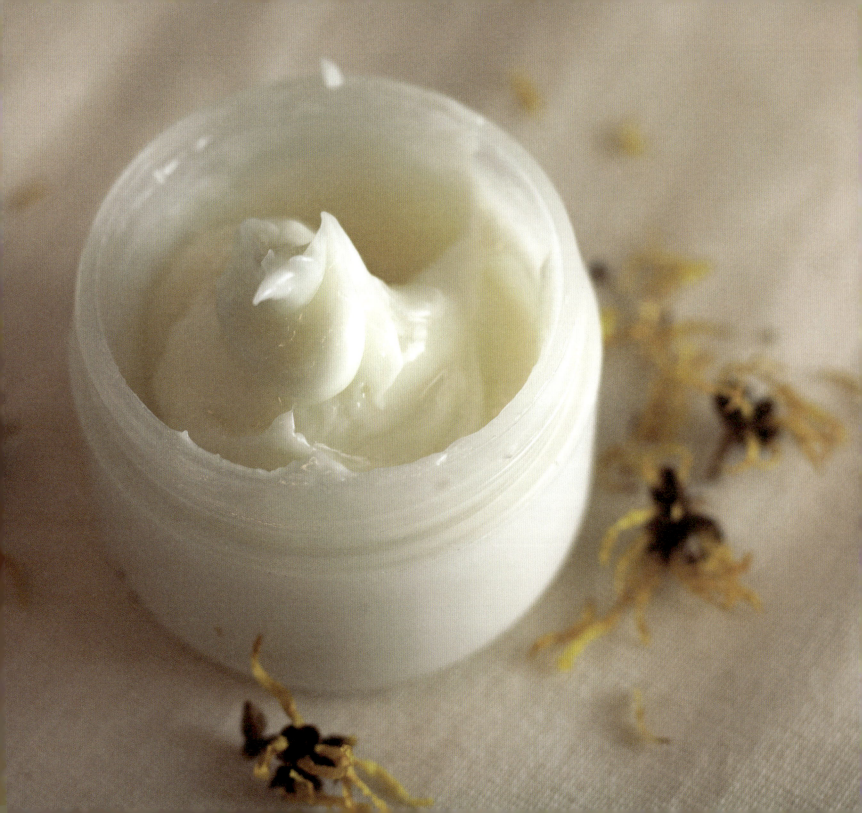

III.
FROZEN WINTER BLOOM CREAM

Applied topically, this refreshingly fragrant witch hazel water-based formulation is a soothing, anti-inflammatory, antiseptic cream. It may be used for minor cutaneous cuts, grazes and irritations, and yet is gentle enough to impart a calming clarity to the complexion through its mildly astringent, cleansing and toning properties. It is one of our most simple creams and is made with just three pure ingredients, intended to be stored as frozen cubes. It is without preservatives of any kind and is an absolute herbology favourite!

Frozen winter bloom cream is so named in reference to the exquisite 'winter bloom' witch hazels (*Hamamelis mollis*) that flower in the Garden during the depths of winter, although (ironically!) they are not the witch hazel ingredient from which the cream is made. The recipe we use calls for witch hazel water, readily sourced from local pharmacies but distilled from *Hamamelis virginiana*.

Although our winter blooming witch hazels are a precious joy for the senses with their saffron-like petals and distinctive fragrance that invigorates the frosty winter air, they are a relatively recent addition to the Garden and would have reached Edinburgh's shores too late to be a feature of the *Materia medica* found in the physic garden of 1670. The 'true' medicinal witch hazels used to make the distilled waters of later English pharmacopoeias and the bottled over-the-counter pharmacy formulation of contemporary times originate from North America.

It is extremely likely that the first witch hazel seeds reached English nurseries by the generous hand of John Bartram, one of the earliest practising Linnaean botanists in North America, sometimes named the 'father of American botany'. Bartram was instrumental in sending seeds from America to gardeners on the continent with whom he was in regular correspondence, and many North American botanicals were first introduced into cultivation in England by this route. Beginning around 1733, Bartram's work was assisted by his association with the English seed merchants.

Beyond the endearing benevolence of kindly fellows such as Bartram, witch hazels have their own highly effective method of ensuring their seed dispersal reaches far and wide: they explode from their ripened capsules with tremendous (ballistic) velocity, demonstrating one of nature's most effective propulsion mechanisms – hence the common name, 'snapping hazel'. The 'witch' in 'witch hazel' in this case doesn't refer to a practitioner of magic but rather originates from the old English *wice* (later *wiche*), which means 'pliable' or 'easy to bend'.

In the indigenous herbal healing traditions of North America, the leaf and bark of the *Hamamelis virginiana* were used to make minor wound-healing remedies, which would be astringent, cooling and antiseptic. *Hamamelis* is high in polyphenolic compounds, tannins and flavonoids, and also holds a very distinctive essential oil. Nowadays, a translucent, ethanol-preserved solution known as witch hazel water is prepared from a steam-distillation of the leaf, bark or twiglets of *Hamamelis virginiana* – it has the distinctive fragrance of the essential oil but with no tannins present. Witch hazel water is the quintessential ingredient for the recipe that follows.

Author's note: *Before you begin, it is recommended that you sterilise all the equipment being used – ice cube tray, measuring jugs and spoons, bowls, whisk, etc. – with boiling water. Air dry them completely.*

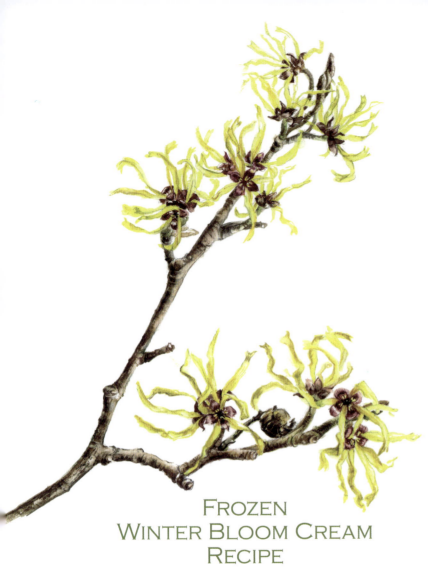

Frozen
Winter Bloom Cream
Recipe

Ingredients

80ml base oil (e.g. almond oil)

1½ heaped tbsp beeswax

40ml witch hazel water

Optional: 1 tsp emulsifying wax
(this helps the mixture 'meld' together)

How to Make

- Put the oil and beeswax into a heatproof bowl
- Pour the distilled witch hazel water into a second bowl
- Place both bowls into a heavy-bottomed pan of shallow water to create a bain-marie
- Heat the pan on the stove until the water is simmering gently
- Wait until the beeswax has melted into the oil and the witch hazel water is warm
- Remove from the heat and lift both bowls carefully out of the pan
- Trickle the witch hazel water slowly into the oil/beeswax solution while stirring rapidly
- Whip the mixture vigorously until it thickens to form a soft cream
- Leave to cool for five minutes
- Spoon the mixture into ice cube trays (1 tsp per cube)
- Put the ice cube trays in the freezer until the mixture is frozen

How to Use

Defrost a cube of mixture, as needed, in a refrigerator overnight for use the next day.

Storage

The frozen cubes may be transferred into a freezer box for storage, if preferred. Remove one cube as required and allow to defrost in a glass jar suitable for cosmetic creams. Once removed from the freezer, the cubes should be used within a fortnight.

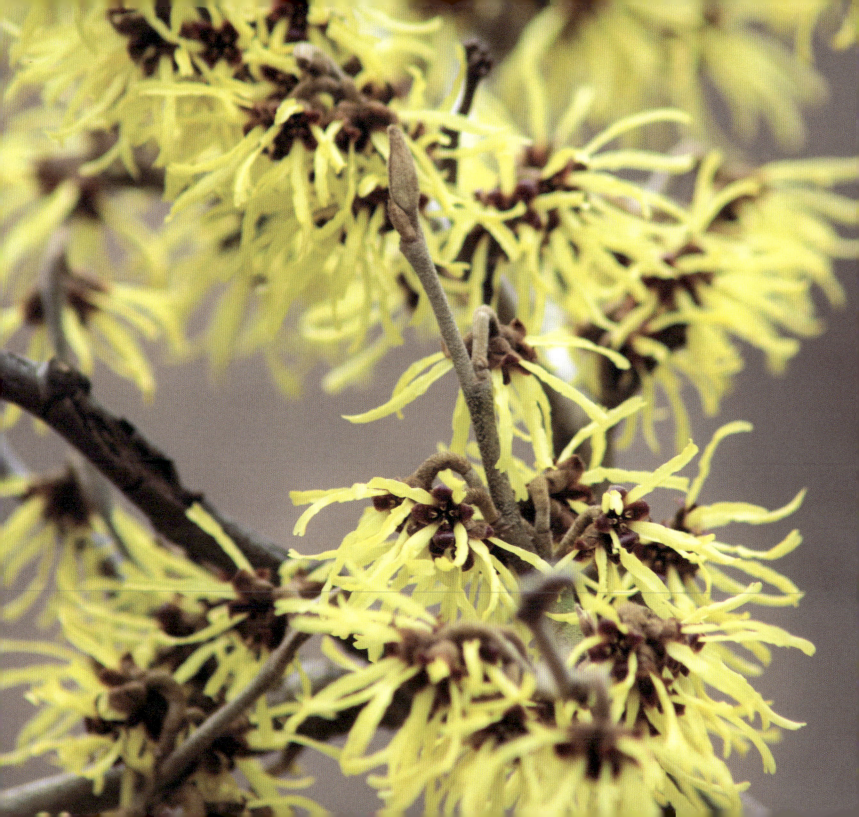

IV.
FIGGY-ORANGE COMPOTE

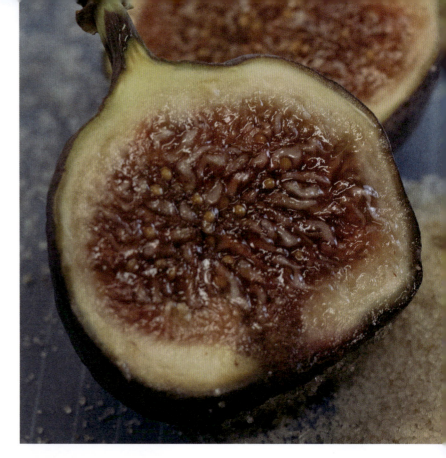

A s the first figgy-orange compote gently bubbled on the hob during one rather late-running herbology evening class many years ago, it was generally agreed that the sweet, orange-spiced aroma that emanated from its cooking pot was deliciously good – something so deeply comforting and wonderful as to be still fondly remembered.

Except for vanilla, all the ingredients for this warming, nutritive and aromatic compote may be found within the *Materia medica* of the old *Edinburgh Pharmacopoeia* (1699), although it is the bitter orange (*Citrus aurantium*) rather than the sweet orange (*Citrus sinensis*) that is included as the medicinal. More contemporary herbals appear equally appreciative of both the sweet and bitter Seville orange, with a particular reference to the peel, oil and juice of the fruits and their constituent flavonoids (most notably hesperidin), volatile principles and vitamin C. Preparations of orange are quintessentially aromatic and carminative digestives that can help to ward off infection.

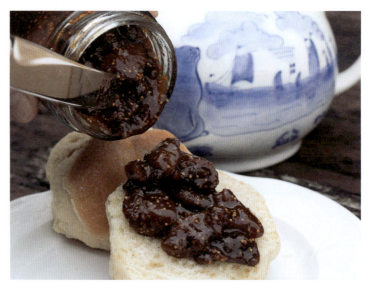

Figs were a feature of the original Edinburgh Physic Garden of 1670 (and happily remain within the current Garden's neighbouring boundaries – espaliered upon one of its nearby nursery walls). With the ability of these nourishing, demulcent, antioxidant fruits to gently tone the alimentary tract, their traditional use in laxative formulations (such as syrup of figs) is quite well known! The recipe that follows, however, should only be mildly aperient….

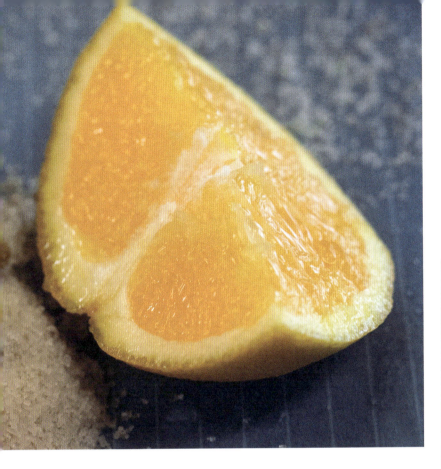

Figgy-Orange Compote Recipe

Ingredients

150g dried whole figs

125ml cold water

1 sweet orange (juice and zest)

½ tsp Ceylon cinnamon powder
(or another spice of your choice)

1 tbsp soft brown sugar

1 tsp vanilla essence

How to Make

- Remove the woody stalks from the figs and cut into smaller pieces, if preferred
- Mix water, orange juice and zest, cinnamon, brown sugar and vanilla in a pan
- Place over a gentle heat and stir until the sugar has dissolved
- Add the figs
- Simmer until figs soften and become plump (approx. ten minutes)
- Remove from heat and allow to cool
- Pour into jars

How to Take

Best enjoyed on cold winter afternoons, topping hot buttered scones or with a little natural yoghurt.

Storage

This recipe stores well for several weeks in the fridge and may be reheated.

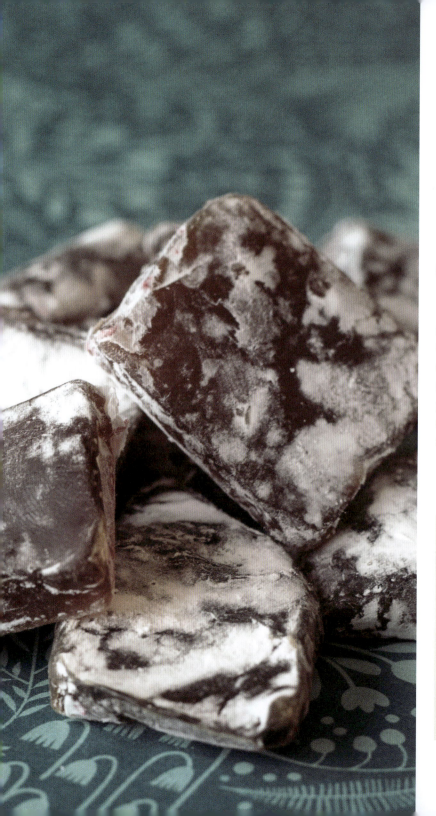

V.

BONFIRE GINGER ROOT TOFFEE

These deliciously good, all-natural ginger chews are the perfect winter walk accompaniment, guaranteed to send a palpable warmth diffusing throughout the body that will reach and rekindle even the most distant and cold of extremities! Ginger has been renowned since ancient times for the carminative comfort it brings to the digestive system and is especially noted nowadays for its more broadly systemic anti-inflammatory properties. Its invigoratingly fiery gingerols add an excellent decongestant and expectorant component into the mix – these little herbal candies are so much more than just a sweetie.

RECIPE

INGREDIENTS

3–4 tbsp ginger root
(freshly and finely grated)

500ml cold water

85g honey
(for a vegan ginger toffee, replace the honey with an equal amount of sugar)

150g raw cane sugar

Cornflour (or icing sugar/tapioca starch) to dust the finished mixture and toffees

HOW TO MAKE

- Decoct the ginger root and water in a small pan (see p. 46 or, if in haste, a ginger syrup from the health food store may be used in place of the decoction)

- Allow the mixture to boil gently until around one cup of liquid remains

- Strain out the ginger root pieces and return the ginger decoction to the pan

- Add the honey and sugar and bring it to the boil once again

- Stir until the sugar has dissolved and reduce the heat to a low simmer

- Allow the decoction to simmer until it reaches the 'hard-ball' stage of candy making (125–130°C/260–265°F on a sugar thermometer)

- Once ready, pour the mixture onto a tray covered with greaseproof paper. Don't spread – let it settle naturally and find its own equilibrium

- Leave to cool for at least 30 minutes

- Once cool, dust the surface with cornflour before peeling it off the greaseproof paper – it should peel off the paper easily in one gloriously satisfying big, pliable piece!

- Turn it over and dust the other side with cornflour

- Cut into sweetie-sized pieces with a sharp, cornflour-dusted knife

- Dust each piece with more cornflour

- Wrap the individual toffees in a small piece of greaseproof paper or dust with a final (liberal) coat of cornflour to stop them sticking together

HOW TO TAKE

These are definitely something to have tucked deep into your pocket on a cold winter walk.

STORAGE

Store in an airtight tin in a cool place for up to eight weeks, or in the fridge for up to four months.

Author's note: *If you don't have a sugar thermometer, you can use the jam-maker's good old drop-in-cold-water technique to gauge whether the mixture is ready. To do this, simply drop a teaspoon of the mixture into a cup of ice-cold water. If it forms a blob that holds its shape out of the water and remains firm when pressed between the fingers, it's ready.*

VI.
WINTER EVERGREEN BUNDLES

These winter botanical bundles are not something that would have been found in the *Edinburgh Pharmacopoeia* at all. However, the aromatic evergreens from which they may be made are among its more arboreal *Materia medica*, most notably in the forms of the resins of various pines, including our native Scots pine (*Pinus sylvestris*), cypress and juniper, whose remedial effects would be achieved through rather more complex means than the creative activity about to be described here. Although arguably, some of the desired end results could be similar, given that the handling of medicinal evergreens and the inhalation of their intoxicating resinous scent is invariably a deeply holistic experience, for both the medicine makers themselves and the recipients of their remedies – or in this case, bundles!

When the earth tilts on its axis in relation to the sun and we reach the zenith of the Winter Solstice darkness in our northern hemisphere, the evergreens become even more noticeable and precious. They are for us – just as they were for our pagan ancestors – symbols of hope and enduring life.

The very presence of evergreens when all else seems faded and passed, fills the heart with faith, for here held safe within these hardy botanicals, our wild and garden 'friends of winter', is the promise of light and warmth being returned to the earth.

We wanted to share the making of these 'winter evergreen bundles' as they were for many years an invigoratingly fragrant fixture of the more 'arts and craft' side of our winter herbology programme. Many of the most fragrant evergreens we have been allowed to use for these bundles were often gathered (with special permission and privilege) from among the Garden's living collection. These include such exotics as the blue Himalayan pine (or Bhutan pine, *Pinus wallichiana*), the Californian incense cedar (*Calocedrus decurrens*) and the weeping juniper tree (*Juniperus flaccida*) that formerly occupied the lawns in front of the Garden's Caledonian Hall.

Originally, these bundles took their inspiration from a beautiful Hopi smudge stick that was kindly gifted as a handling resource for our herbology classes several years ago. The precious botanicals still bound within its loosening threads remain sweetly fragrant and include juniper and its berries.

However, this is a sacred object, of sacred herbs and smoke rituals, all of which belong to the First Nations peoples and their indigenous culture rather than our own. So, while the structural form and creative thread work of the original smudge stick has influenced how our winter evergreen bundles are made, it is not our intention that something so sacred is in any way appropriated.

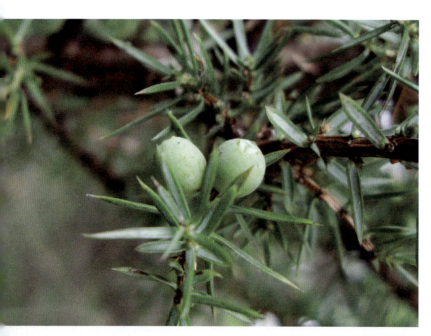

WINTER EVERGREEN BUNDLES

INGREDIENTS & EQUIPMENT

Aromatic evergreen cuttings, e.g. pine, cedar, juniper (how much you collect depends on the abundance of your botanical source, how many bundles you wish to make and how you intend to use them. Small 18–30cm-long pieces are required for incense sticks)

Small garden hand clippers to cut the evergreens as you work

An old pair of gardening gloves (a robust leather or suede will afford the best protection for your hands – some of the botanicals we have worked with in the past, and those recommended above, have been found to be rather prickly but are absolutely worth the effort!)

Thin but sturdy thread or twine (embroidery yarn is good – different colours may be used to code the evergreens and remind you of what is in your bundle)

A page of newspaper folded in half, or a 30 × 45cm soft piece of cloth

HOW TO MAKE

- Gather a few of the evergreen cuttings
- Arrange the cuttings in a bundle
- Tie together in a decorative way using threads or slender ribbons
- The bundles may be hung or displayed as festive ornaments

Author's note: *We suggest that our bundles be kept and enjoyed as aromatic artefacts only.*

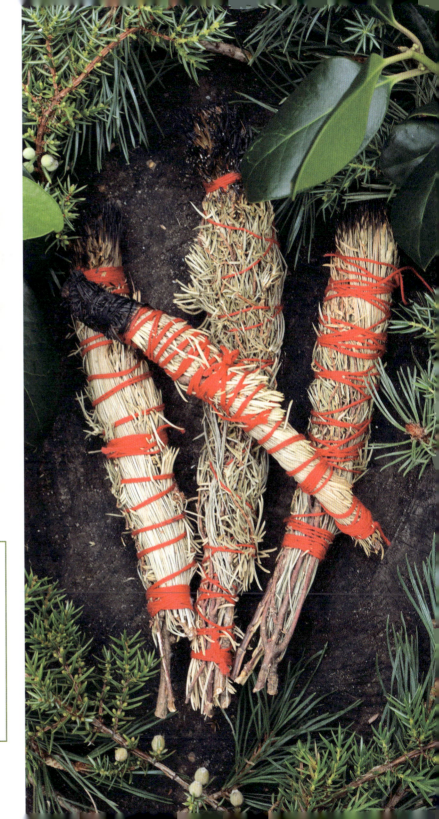

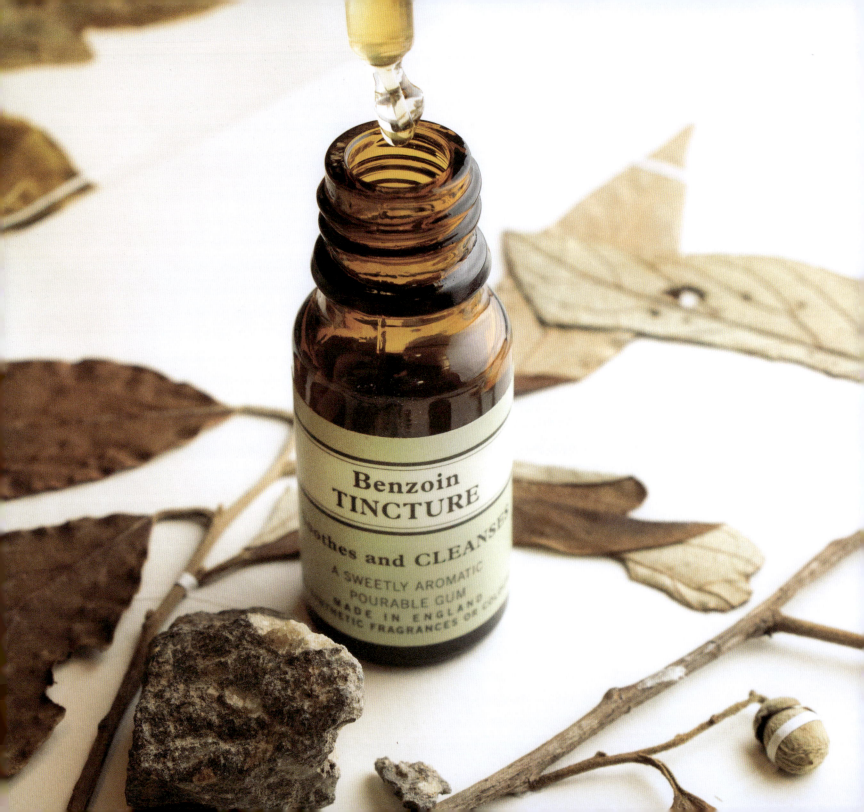

VII.

GUMS, RESINS, RUBS & VAPOURS

EMBROCATIONS & LINIMENTS

The very words 'embrocation and liniment' seem to conjure something of the spirit that must have emanated from within the old herbal dispensaries of Culpeper's time and lingered well into the 20th century at places such as Duncan Napier's of Edinburgh. Indeed, such were the remedies that would have appeared in the extract-stained and well-annotated pages of a bygone pharmaceutical codex, among all the other staples of pharmacy for the practising apothecary and later herbalist.

Essentially the same, embrocation and liniment both describe various medicinal rubbing lotions that nowadays are almost indistinguishable; they were, however, traditionally regarded as rather different remedies.

A liniment (*linimentum*, meaning 'to anoint') generally refers to a warming liquid or semi-fluid preparation that is used topically. Liniments are usually solutions of already prepared extracts that hold aromatic compounds like methyl salicylate, benzoin resin, menthol and capsaicin. These mildly analgesic, rubefacient, sedative or stimulating substances are dissolved in a lubricating lipid base (e.g. a vulnerary herb-infused oil), or a mixture of alcoholic tincture (which evaporates as it is warmed on the body) and oil, so that they are more penetrative. Sometimes vinegar may be used, with the addition of a few drops of essential oil to enhance the effect.

Liniments may occasionally be applied locally with a soft cloth, but they are generally rubbed into the body in slow circular movements for deeper integumentary tissue stimulation. Liniments are excellent topical remedies for the relief of muscular discomfort, stiffness, cramps, rheumatic agues, bruises, strains and sprains, etc.

An embrocation is generally an oil-based liniment only, more often in the past used as a pectoral remedy to ease respiratory congestion and bronchial troubles. Eucalyptus, menthol and/or camphorated oils were once popular ingredients of childhood embrocations.

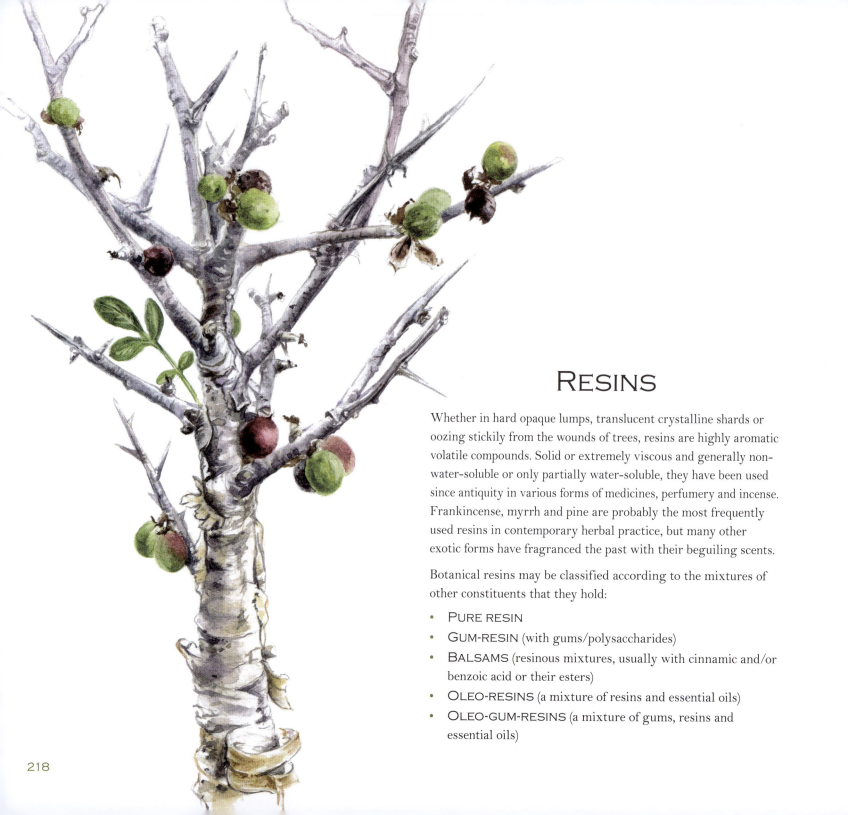

Resins

Whether in hard opaque lumps, translucent crystalline shards or oozing stickily from the wounds of trees, resins are highly aromatic volatile compounds. Solid or extremely viscous and generally non-water-soluble or only partially water-soluble, they have been used since antiquity in various forms of medicines, perfumery and incense. Frankincense, myrrh and pine are probably the most frequently used resins in contemporary herbal practice, but many other exotic forms have fragranced the past with their beguiling scents.

Botanical resins may be classified according to the mixtures of other constituents that they hold:

- PURE RESIN
- GUM-RESIN (with gums/polysaccharides)
- BALSAMS (resinous mixtures, usually with cinnamic and/or benzoic acid or their esters)
- OLEO-RESINS (a mixture of resins and essential oils)
- OLEO-GUM-RESINS (a mixture of gums, resins and essential oils)

THE BENEFITS OF BENZOIN

Benzoin is one of nature's finest oleo-gum resins, and from among all its worldly virtues (perfumery and cosmetics), it is probably most noted as an exemplary antiseptic, anti-inflammatory and expectorant compound. It's most effective as an ingredient of cough mixtures, topical chest rubs and steam vapour inhalations.

As a vapour remedy, benzoin is unsurpassed, and what better way is there to enjoy such a deeply aromatic and spirit-soothing medicine than quite simply to just breathe it in? One of the reasons benzoin works so well as a steam vapour inhalant is that (being an oleo-gum-resin) it is relatively soluble in water – especially hot water.

A pourable benzoin oil, tincture of benzoin, or friar's balsam mixed with hot water (as directed on the bottle) are all excellent for this purpose and for ease of use may still be found in some local pharmacies or, more likely, the herbal suppliers listed at the beginning of this book (p. 23).

I can only describe the pharmacy-sourced benzoin oil (mobile), with its deeply resonant and balsam-like aroma, as alluring. Others point to its vanilla top notes with warm hints of chocolate. However you interpret its fragrance, it has the consistency of sticky molasses and a tantalisingly slow drip as it exudes from the bottle.

It is recommended that if these truly headier scents of the medicinal resinous compounds have not been adequately captured during the extraction and/or infusion methodologies given here, a few additional drops of the oil will do the trick, and only enhance the overall therapeutic experience that ensues.

The following remedies are intended for topical use as soothing, respiratory and nasal passageway decongestants, to comfort the bronchioles and ease the breathing difficulties of chesty coughs and colds. Apply topically at night – rub in slowly and thoroughly and then take several deep breaths….

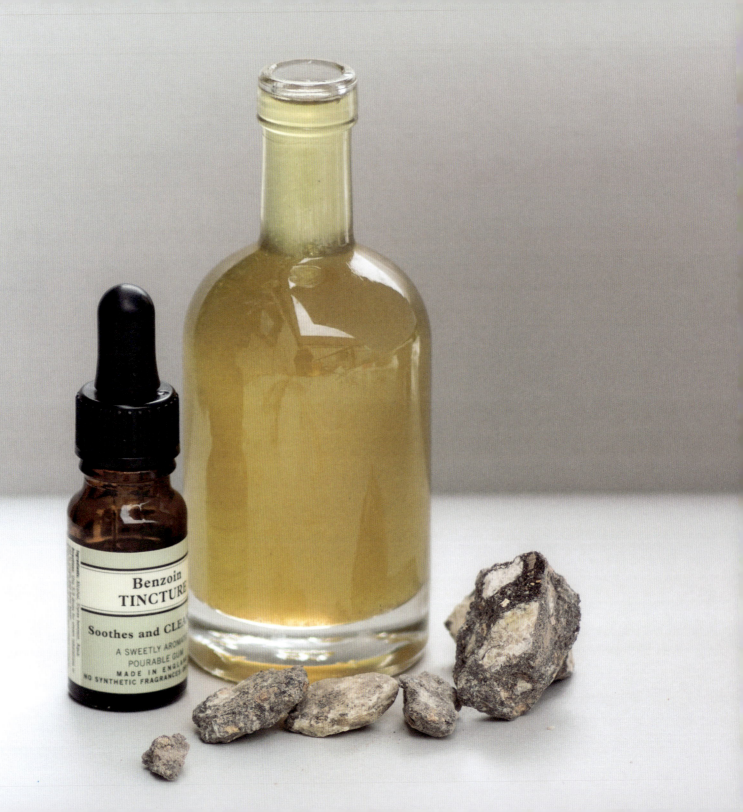

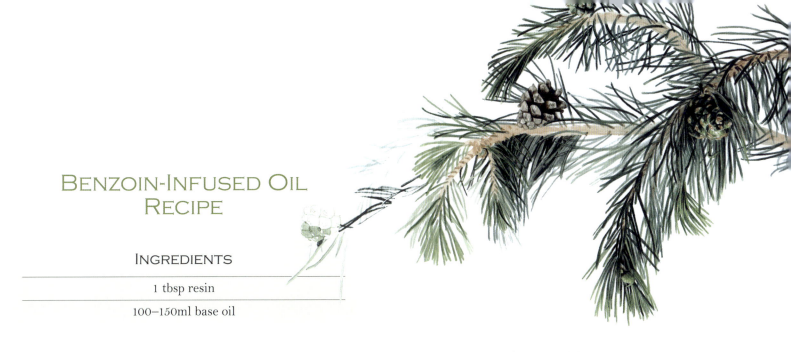

BENZOIN-INFUSED OIL RECIPE

INGREDIENTS

1 tbsp resin

100–150ml base oil

HOW TO MAKE

- Grind the resin to a fine powder (if the resin is gooey, freeze it and grind while still frozen)
- Pour the powdered resin into a heatproof screw-top jar (dedicated for this purpose)
- Add base oil (the amount can be varied according to requirements)
- Shake vigorously
- Place the jar in a bain-marie and warm gently on the hob for at least one hour
- Remove the jar from the bain-marie and dry it off
- Put the jar in a warm place (ideally on top of an Aga stove or near a fireplace that is frequently hot!)
- Allow the oil to infuse for several weeks, shaking frequently and vigorously
- Once the oil is intoxicatingly aromatic, it's ready!
- Strain out any undissolved particles of resin
- Bottle (dark amber glass is best) and label

HOW TO USE

Not for oral consumption. Apply topically just as it is, as a soothing emollient, mildly antiseptic and anti-inflammatory remedy ideal for uncomplicated (closed) slow-to-heal wounds and on minor irritations of the cutaneous tissues. Or incorporate into the embrocation/liniment recipe that follows.

STORAGE

Store in a cool, dark place for up to a year.

Author's note: *Always sample a little of any topical formulation before more liberal use. This is especially important with oleo-gum-resins of a balsamic nature, like benzoin. Benzoin essential oil holds benzoic and cinnamic acids – avoid use where there is a known allergy. Do not use over an extended period or diffuse. Do not apply over expansive areas of the body or use in remedies for children under five.*

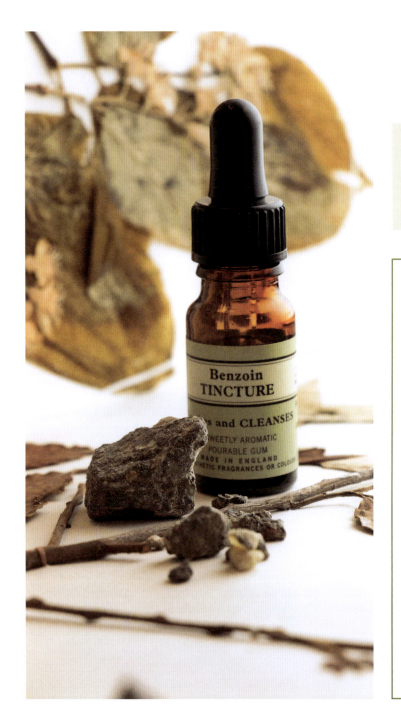

Alcoholic Extract of Benzoin Recipe

Ingredients

1 part resin

3 parts pure alcohol (minimum of 40% strength – we recommend vodka)

How to Make

- Grind the resin to a fine powder
- Start by using small amounts to create a sample
- Pour the powdered resin into a screw-top jar (dedicated for this purpose)
- Add the alcohol
- Allow to steep for several weeks and shake vigorously throughout
- Strain out any remaining sediments of undissolved resin through a piece of muslin
- Bottle (dark amber glass is best) and label
- Dilute with the oil before use

How to Use

Not for oral consumption. Use in topical formulations, liniments and/or embrocations.

Storage

If stored in a cool, dark place, alcoholic gum-resin extracts of this sort will keep for several years.

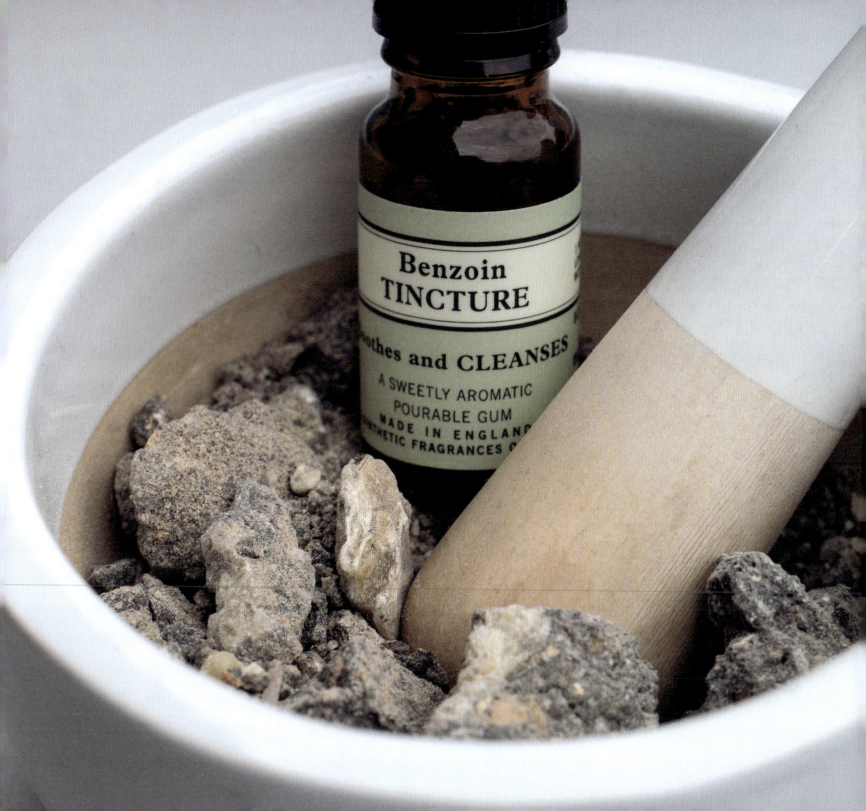

Benzoin
TINCTURE

...othes and CLEANSES

A SWEETLY AROMATIC
POURABLE GUM

MADE IN ENGLAND

...NTHETIC FRAGRANCES O...

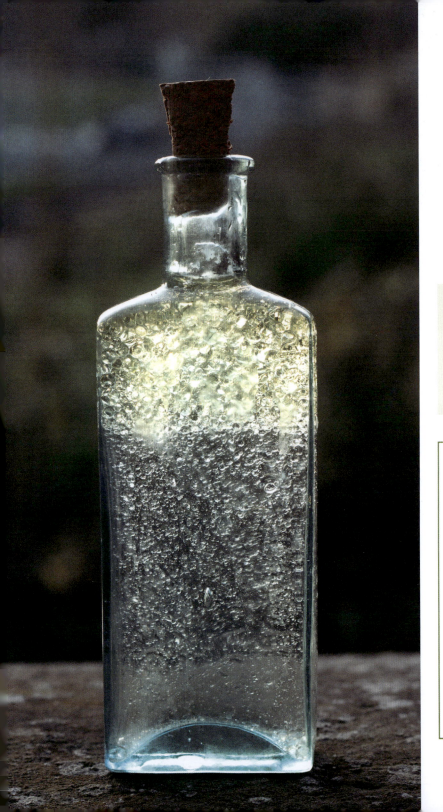

OIL OF BENZOIN EMBROCATION RECIPE

INGREDIENTS

50ml (10 tsp) of base oil (e.g. pure almond or benzoin-infused oil, p. 221)

3–5 drops benzoin (resinoid)

Essential oil (pharmacy formulation)

HOW TO MAKE

- Mix base oil with benzoin oil
- Pour into a small bottle or jar, lid and label

HOW TO USE

Not for oral consumption. Warm the oil gently in the bottle or jar before use. Rub a small amount gently over the chest, following a warm bath, before bed, and breathe in the vapours deeply.

STORAGE

If stored in a cool, dark place, a simple embrocation like this should keep for up to a year.

OIL OF BENZOIN LINIMENT RECIPE

INGREDIENTS

1 part (e.g. 50ml) benzoin-infused oil

1 part (e.g. 50ml) benzoin alcoholic extract

10–12 drops of benzoin essential oil
(a resinoid pharmacy formulation)

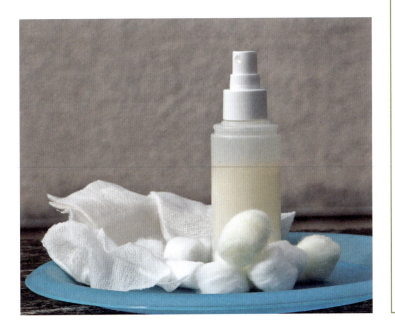

HOW TO MAKE

- Place the ingredients in a bottle – ideally one with a spritz nozzle
- Shake vigorously to encourage the formulations to blend (they will naturally separate on standing)

HOW TO USE

Not for oral consumption. Warm and shake well before use. Pour a small amount into your cupped hand or spritz a little where required and rub in.

STORAGE

If stored in a cool, dark place, a simple liniment of this sort should keep for up to a year.

Author's note: *Do not exceed around one eighth the number of drops of essential oil to millilitres of liquid used in any liniment formulation of this sort (e.g. 1–5 drops essential oil to 40ml liquid). Handle essential oils with care and only add one drop at a time, blending thoroughly and sampling before adding more.*

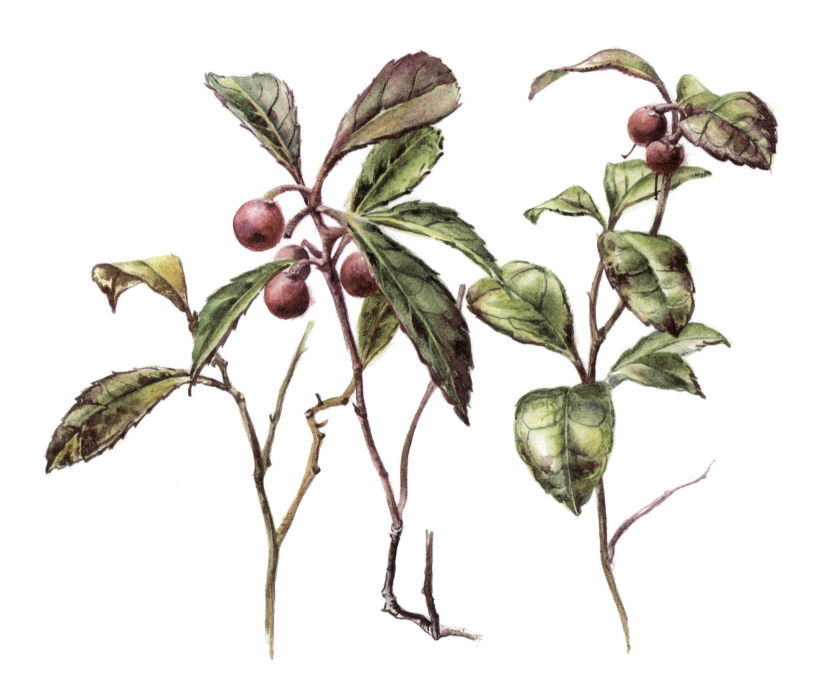

BENZOIN VAPOUR RUB
RECIPE

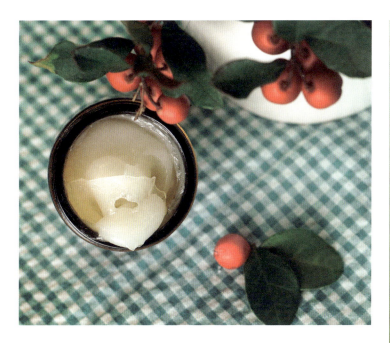

For deep overnight inhalation of warm benzoin vapours, this soft rub is a wonderfully soothing, sleep-inducing, breathe-easy formulation to use whenever you have a chesty cough or cold. It can be easily adapted too – try a pine resin-infused oil or eucalyptus and menthol essential oils.

INGREDIENTS

50ml benzoin resin-infused oil (see p. 221)
3 tsp beeswax
5–10 drops benzoin (resinoid) essential oil (pharmacy formulation)

HOW TO MAKE

- Warm the oil in a bain-marie
- Melt the beeswax into the oil
- Once the wax has liquefied, remove from the hob
- Add the essential oil drops
- Stir through thoroughly
- Pour into an ointment jar
- Allow to cool, lid and label

HOW TO USE

Use at night in bed – smooth a small amount over the chest and throat and a little just in front of and around the lobes of both ears.

STORAGE

Store in a cool, dark place for up to a year.

Author's note: *An alternative embrocation, liniment and vapour rub could be made using oil of wintergreen and alcoholic extract of wintergreen* (Gaultheria procumbens). *Wintergreen has its own very distinctive character and noted phenolic compounds but may be used for its similarly highly antiseptic, anti-inflammatory, mildly analgesic and – most noticeably – antirheumatic properties. Wintergreen essential oil consists almost entirely of methyl salicylate – avoid in asthma or where there is a known salicylate allergy.*

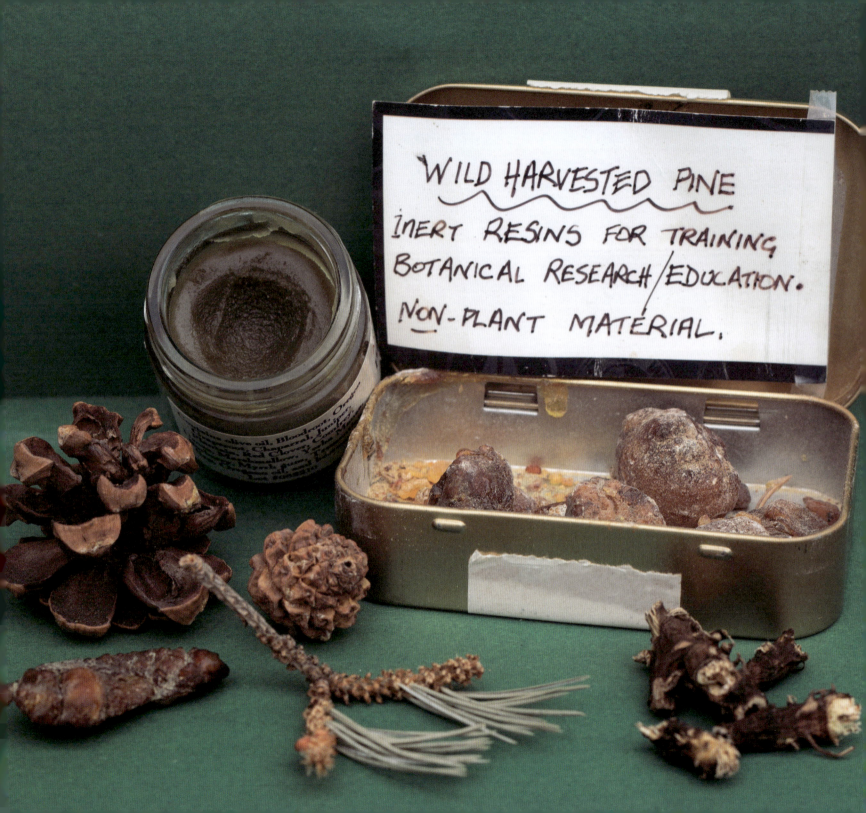

WILD HARVESTED PINE
INERT RESINS FOR TRAINING
BOTANICAL RESEARCH/EDUCATION.
NON-PLANT MATERIAL.

VIII.
PINE RESIN SALVE

Here's a contemporary take on an old pine resin remedy that shared a place in the home pharmacy of the Highlands and Islands, as well as across the plains of the American Midwest.

The key ingredient for each formulation is the resin sourced from local pines – the Scots pine (*Pinus sylvestris*) and piñon pine (*Pinus edulis*) – the latter being one of the most prominent trees of northern New Mexico, responsible in no small part to the unique scent of the air around places such as Taos and Santa Fe. It is from here, almost every year, that we have received a small, eagerly anticipated gift of piñon pine resin, carefully gathered and packaged by one of our distant herbology friends. The piñon pine resin is a sacred resin commonly used by First Nations peoples, so this is regarded as among our most precious *Materia medica*.

In the Highlands and Islands, original recipes for pine resin salve used beeswax, hog's lard and the resin from various pines to make either a simple healing ointment for boils and sores or an antiseptic plaster, while the traditional indigenous pine pitch salve has a reputation for assisting in the removal of splinters and thorns. Both remedies, dependent upon the concentration of resin used, induce warm and stimulating rubefacient effects that help to 'draw things out' and as such are excellent remedies for gardeners to have to hand.

A very satisfying pine resin salve may be prepared from the resins that exude naturally from storm-fallen branches of pines, and winter is the ideal time to gather resin from these – especially as it will be hardened by the colder temperatures, making it easier to collect. An old knife is perfect for collecting the resin, which may be carefully scraped free. Even if hardened on the outside, a resin lump is still likely to be soft and sticky at its core, so collect it on a piece of well-waxed paper or in a dedicated resin-collecting tin or jar.

Author's note: *Whenever gathering pine resin, never pull it off the healing wound of a living tree as it is effectively the tree's bandage. If some resin is dripping further down the trunk, past the wounded area, it may be gently removed from there. In warmer times, 'blisters' of resin form on some pines and these may be 'popped'. From wherever you gather your resin, do so with love and gratitude.*

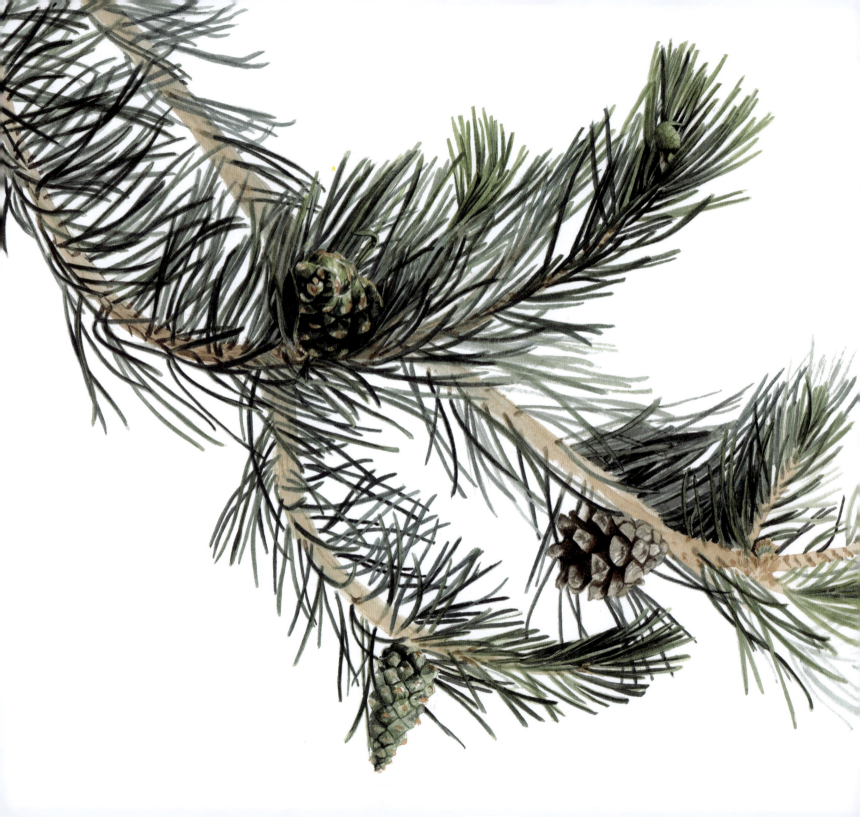

Pine Resin Salve Recipe

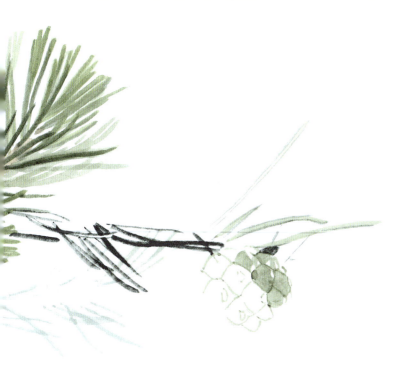

Ingredients

50ml pure base oil

½ tsp pine resin

1½ tsp beeswax

How to Make

- Pour the desired amount of base oil into a glass jam jar
- Place the jar into a bain-marie and warm the oil through gently
- Once the oil is quite hot, add the pine resin in small lumps
- Allow the resin to dissolve as thoroughly as possible into the oil
- Once the pine resin has completely liquefied, add the beeswax
- Allow the beeswax to melt into the warm pine oil solution
- Remove the jar from the bain-marie and allow the balm to cool and form
- Lid and label your jar with the date and ingredients used

How to Use

Apply topically as needed to grazes, sores or slow-to-heal wounds.

Storage

Store in a cool, dry place in dark amber glass jars. Stored this way, it should last for up to a year.

Author's note: *An alternative and yet therapeutically similar recipe would use bee gum balm – an exemplary healing ointment.*

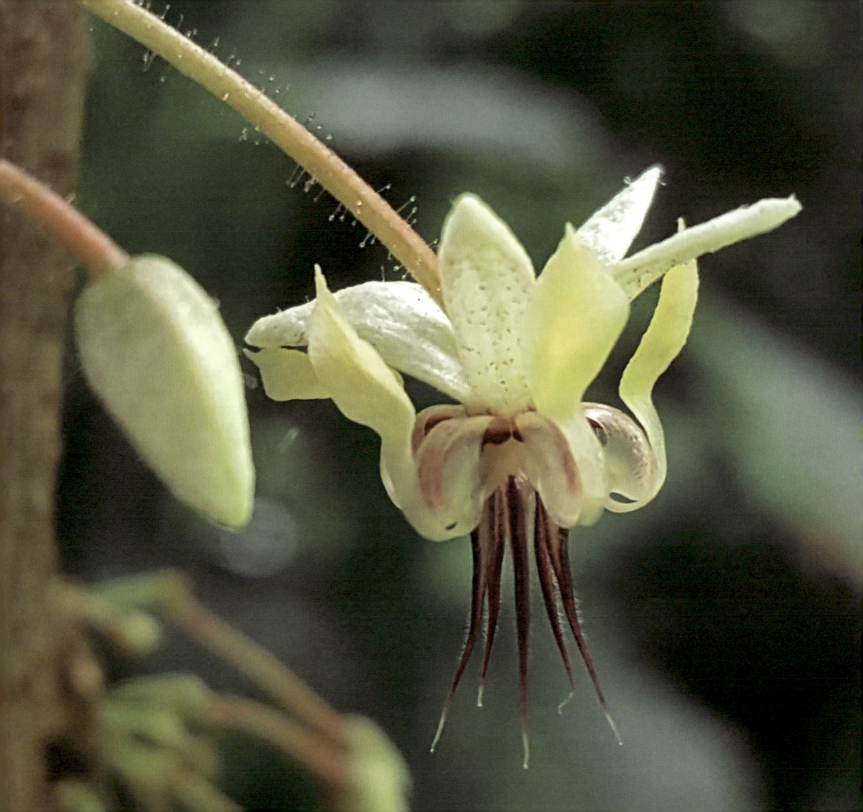

IX.
RAW CACAO TRUFFLES

The cauliflorous fruits and the pale flower clusters of the cocoa tree (*Theobroma cacao*) are almost lost among all the other luxuriant foliage in the humid realm of one of the Garden's tropical glasshouses, but they are there, waiting to be found. The discovery of one (or usually several) of the bean-bearing pods, at whatever stage of their ripeness – and the beautiful beans themselves, nestled together closely as they are inside the pod's soft white pulp – is a genuine pleasure.

In its natural equatorial range, the cocoa tree blooms the whole year round and its flowers and pods may be seen on the tree at the same time. Over a half-year period, thousands of delicate flowers adorn the trunk and branches of the cacao tree, but only a few of these will eventually develop into pods and each flower blooms for only a single day – its bud begins to open in the afternoon, the emerging petals unfurling throughout the night into full bloom by early morning.

Chocolate is a natural energy enhancer, and our recipe for raw cacao truffles makes the most of chocolate's nutritional as well as medicinal (nutraceutical) nature. Each little bean is jam-packed full of goodness. Raw cacao holds an absolutely outstanding number of minerals and trace elements (including magnesium, calcium, iron, zinc, potassium, sulphur, phosphorus, manganese, copper and chromium) with vitamins A, B and C (antioxidant polyphenolic compounds).

As if that wasn't sufficient, cocoa also contains all these extraordinary constituents: theobromine (a mood- and energy-enhancing anti-inflammatory, which may also function as a cough suppressant and anti-asthmatic); tryptophan and serotonin (the feel-good hormones); phenethylamine (found in the fermented beans); and anandamide (a compound we produce in our bodies when we fall in love). Anandamide is an endorphin known as the 'bliss molecule' – it apparently binds to the body's cannabinoid receptors and is believed to play a role in producing feelings of happiness and even euphoria. Cocoa and black truffle fungi (*Tuber melanosporum*) are the only botanicals on earth known to hold it.

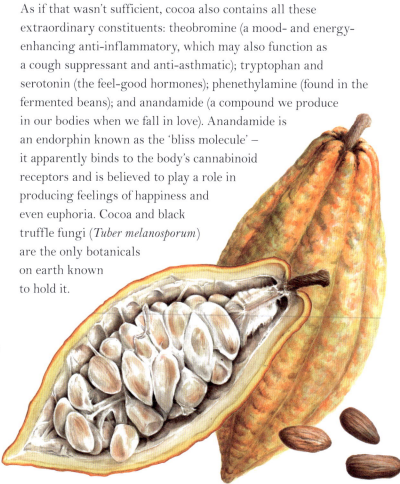

RAW CACAO TRUFFLES RECIPE

INGREDIENTS

10 dates (stones removed)

A handful of chopped pecan nuts
(or nuts/seeds of your choice)

2 tbsp raw cacao powder

1 tbsp coconut flour

1 tbsp coconut water

1½ tsp ground green cardamom powder
(or more if desired)

Optional dusting powders: spice powder blend, beetroot powder, dessicated coconut, rosehip powder, carob powder or dark chocolate powder

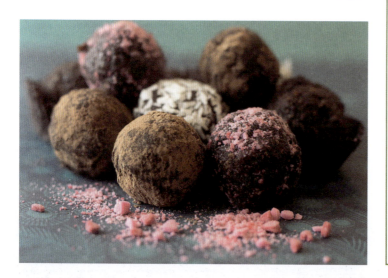

HOW TO MAKE

- Cut the stoned dates into small pieces and blitz in a blender

- Add the pecan nuts, raw cacao powder, coconut flour, coconut water and green cardamom powder, and blitz together in a blender until a thick paste is formed

- Adjust the consistency by adding more cacao powder (to thicken) or coconut water (to soften)

- Roll into small balls and dust in a spice powder blend of your choice

- Alternatively, dust with beetroot powder, desiccated coconut, rosehip powder or delicious carob powder

- Optional: twirl in dark melted chocolate for a truly indulgent, yet nutritiously good and wholesome treat!

HOW TO TAKE

Enjoy one (or several!) around 4pm with a cup of tea to restore flagging energies and depleted blood sugar and help you over that last hump of a hard day – or quite simply whenever you feel you've lost your va-va-voom!

STORAGE

Store in a lidded box in the fridge and consume within a fortnight.

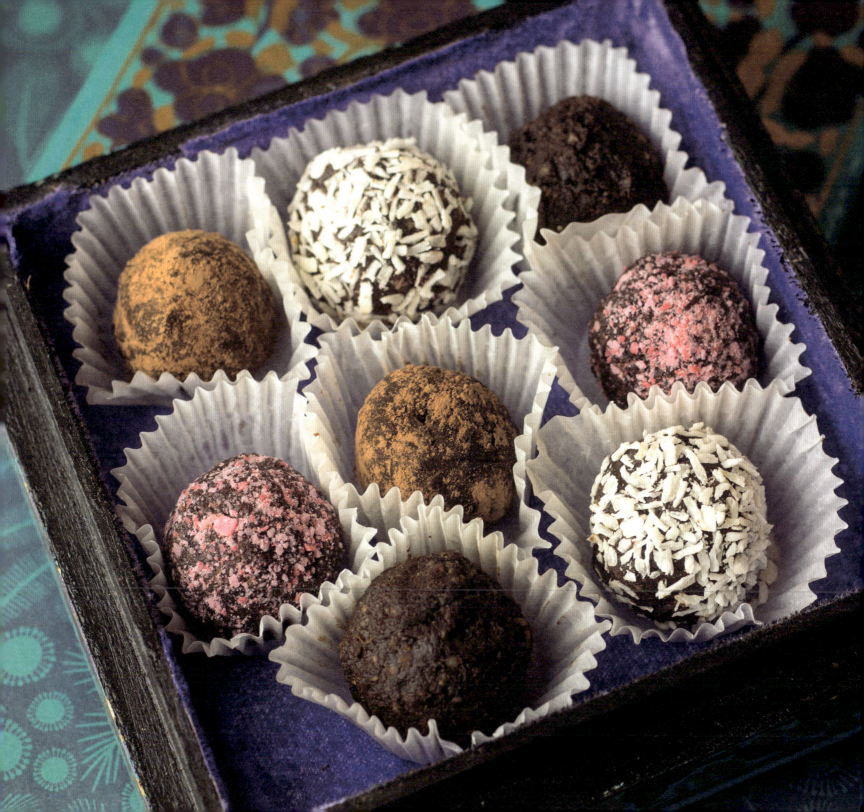

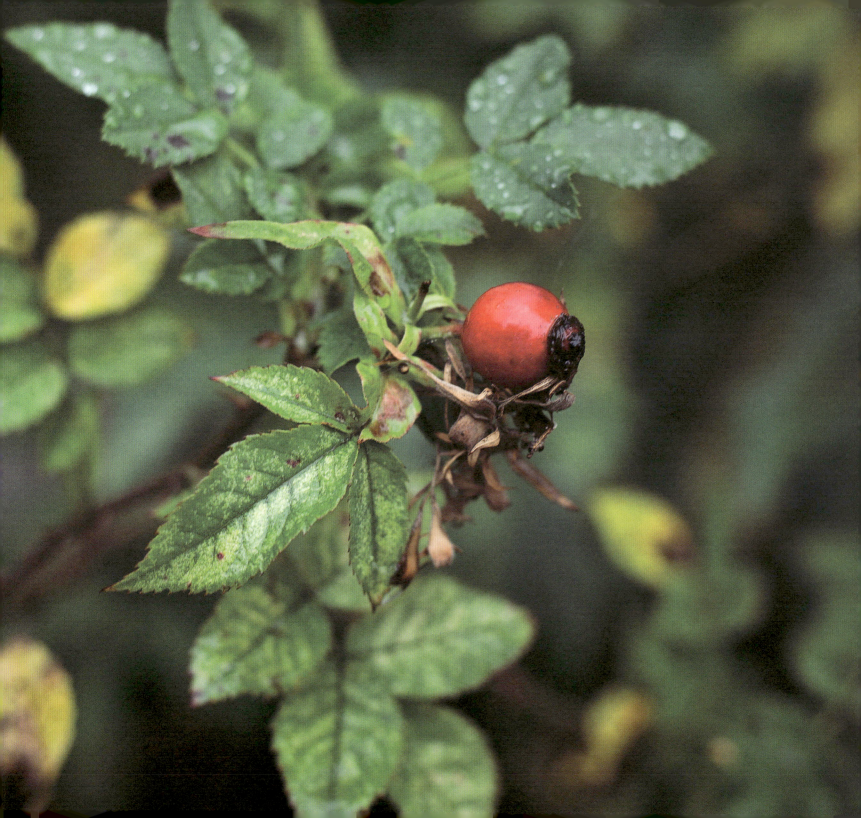

GLOSSARY

ADAPTOGENS

Plants that help your body 'adapt' to stress and restore its natural balance, helping to reduce negative effects

AERIAL PARTS

The parts of a plant that grow above soil, in the air (e.g. the stalk, stem, leaves, fruits and flowers)

AGUE

A fever or fit of shivering

ALEMBICS

Apparatus used for the distillation of liquids

APERIENT

A remedy used to relieve constipation

AURICLES

The visible part of the human ear

BAIN-MARIE

A piece of equipment used to gently heat or melt materials and keep them warm; the name is derived from the French 'bain de Marie', meaning 'Mary's bath'

BELTANE

The Gaelic May Day festival traditionally held on 1 May; Beltane is a Celtic word that means 'fires of Bel'

CAULIFLOROUS

Producing flowers or fruits directly from the stem or branch

CAUSE CÉLÈBRE

A controversial issue, person or event that attracts a great deal of attention

CHARGE

Apply a cover or coat of

CHRONOTROPIC

Influencing the rate of your heartbeat

DISPENSATORY

A book containing the composition, preparation and application of various drugs

---

E.O.

Abbreviation for an 'essential oil'

GALENICALS

Medicinal extracts, named after Claudius Galen, a classical physician and author of ancient Greece

GREEN PHARMACY

The practice of botanical (herbal) medicine making – an alternative, holistic, preventative approach that seeks to reduce potentially harmful impacts of more orthodox pharmaceuticals

---

HYGROSCOPIC

Hygroscopy refers to the phenomenon of attracting and holding onto water molecules. Gels, honey and glycerine/glycerol are hygroscopic.

LINNAEAN BOTANY

Named after Carolus Linnaeus, who is generally regarded as the founder of modern taxonomy and who drew up what are thought to be the first set of rules for assigning names to plants and animals

LUGHNASA
A Gaelic festival marking the beginning of harvest season, historically observed in Scotland, Ireland and the Isle of Man

MANNA
(From the bible) a food from the Gods that saved the Israelites from dying of hunger in the desert

MATERIA MEDICA
A Latin pharmaceutical term applied to the body of collected knowledge about the therapeutic properties of any substance used for healing

MARC
The plant material that is used in making a herbal extraction or preparation

NUTRACEUTICAL
Nourishing compounds with additional medicinal benefits beyond their purely nutritional value

PERSEIDS
Made from tiny space debris from the comet Swift-Tuttle, the Perseid meteor shower is named after the constellation Perseus

PHYSIC GARDEN
A type of herb garden featuring medicinal plants; medieval physic gardens existed by the year 800

POSTPRANDIAL
Occurring after a meal

SAMHAIN
A Gaelic festival on 1 November marking the end of the harvest season and the beginning of winter, which begins on the evening of 31 October

SIMPLE
A herbal remedy consisting of one ingredient only

STILL
Apparatus used for the distillation of liquids

TISANE
A delicate infusion of fresh or dried herbs served hot or cold, usually made from botanical plants

UNGUENT
A soft viscous substance for lubrication that is similar to an ointment

VIBRATIONAL MEDICINE
A form of alternative medicine and therapy that uses energies or vibrational frequencies to help restore or maintain well-being

VOLATILES
Organic compounds that have a high vapour pressure at room temperature

VULNERARY
A herbal remedy used to help heal wounds and inflammation; the word 'vulnerary' comes from the Latin 'vulnus', meaning 'wound'

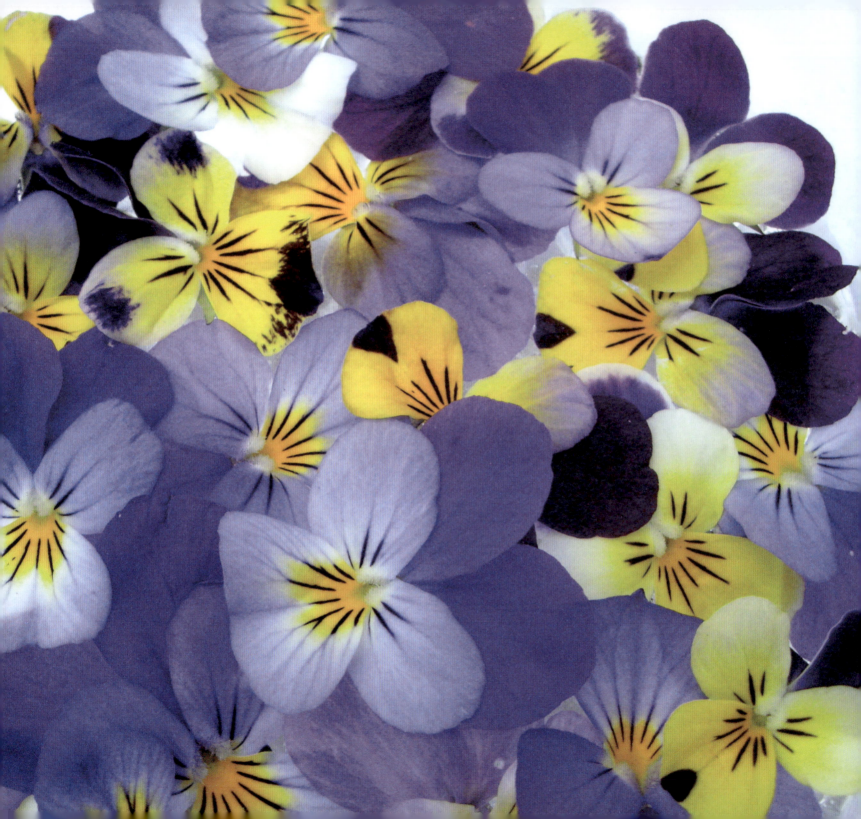

RECOMMENDED READING

This is by no means a complete listing for all the sources consulted for this book but is hopefully a useful starting point for anyone interested in reading more about herbology.

In addition to these titles, an excellent and easily accessible digital library resource for any budding herbologist or medicinal herb researcher alike is the Herbal History Research Network: **https://herbalhistory.org**

A fully digitised version of our edition of Culpeper's *The Complete Herbal* may be found online via the Wellcome Collection: **https://wellcomecollection.org/works/pjvn9c9z/items**

———

Books

ALLEN, D.E., HATFIELD, G., *Medicinal Plants in Folk Tradition: An Ethnobotany of Britain & Ireland*, Timber Press, Cambridge, England, 2004

ATKINSON, T., *Napiers History of Herbal Healing, Ancient & Modern*, Luath Press Limited, Edinburgh, 2003

BARKER, A., *Remembered Remedies: Traditional Scottish Plant Lore*, Birlinn, Edinburgh, 2011

BARTRAM, T., *Encyclopedia of Herbal Medicine*, Grace Publishers, Dorset, England, 1995

BUHNER, S.H., *Sacred Plant Medicine: Explorations in the Practice of Indigenous Herbalism*, Roberts Rinehart Pub., New York, 1996

CRAIG, W.S., *History of the Royal College of Physicians of Edinburgh*, Blackwell Scientific Publications, Oxford, 1976

CULPEPER, N., *The Complete Herbal and English Physician Enlarged*, Thomas Kelly, London, 1846

EVELYN, J. ESQ., *Kalendarium Hortense*, Jo. Martyn and Ja. Allestry, printers to the Royal Society, London, 1664

FLETCHER, H.R., BROWN, W.H., *The Royal Botanic Garden Edinburgh 1670–1970*, Her Majesty's Stationery Office, Edinburgh, 1970

GERARD, J., *The Herbal or General History of Plants: The Complete 1633 Edition as Revised and Enlarged by Thomas Johnson*, Courier Dover Publications, 2015

GREEN, J., *The Herbal Medicine-Maker's Handbook: A Home Manual*, Crossing Press, Berkeley, California, 2000

GRIEVE, M., *A Modern Herbal*, Jonathan Cape, London, 1931

HOFFMAN, D., *The Holistic Herbal*, Findhorn Press, Forres, 1983

HOLMES, P., *The Energetics of Western Herbs*, Artemis Press, Boulder, Colorado, 1989

MILLS, S.Y., *Out of the Earth*, Viking, London, 1991

PASSMORE, R., *Fellows of Edinburgh's College of Physicians during the Scottish Enlightenment*, Royal College of Physicians of Edinburgh, Edinburgh, 2001

PENGELLY, A., *The Constituents of Medicinal Plants: An Introduction to the Chemistry and Therapeutics of Herbal Medicines*, CABI Publishing, London, 2004

REID, J., *The Scot's Gard'ner*, Mainstream Publishing Company, Edinburgh, 1988

RITCHIE, R. P., *The Early Days of The Royal College of Phisitians Edinburgh*, George P. Johnston, Edinburgh, 1899

SUTHERLAND, J., *Hortus Medicus Edinburgensis*, Edinburgh, 1683

TIERRA, M., *Planetary Herbology*, Lotus Press, Santa Fe, 1988

VOGEL, V., *American Indian Medicine*, University of Oklahoma Press, 1970

WOOD, M., *The Earthwise Herbal*, North Atlantic Books, Berkeley, California, 2008

WREN, R.C., *Potter's New Cyclopaedia of Botanical Drugs & Preparations*, The C.W. Daniel Company Limited, Saffron Walden, England, 1994

JOURNALS

Edinburgh Pharmacopoeia, Royal College of Physicians of Edinburgh, Edinburgh, 1699 (Translated by Robert Mill, RBGE Research Associate, for the author, autumn 2019)

Robertson, F.W., 'James Sutherland's "Hortus Medicus Edinburgensis" (1683)' *Garden History*, 29(2): 121–151, 2001

WEBSITES

American Botanical Council, *A Pictorial History of Herbs in Medicine and Pharmacy*, **https://herbalgram.org/resources/herbalgram/issues/42/table-of-contents/article547**

Bee Culture: The Magazine of American Beekeeping, Riddle, S., *The Chemistry of Honey*, **https://beeculture.com/the-chemistry-of-honey**

Cacao Mama, *Nutrition & Science*, **https://cacaomama.com/nutrition-science**

Evolving Magazine, Enos, T., Galiger, E., *Trementia*, **https://evolvingmagazine.com/trementina**

Kitrusy, *Honey-Ginger Chews*, **https://kitrusy.com/ginger-honey-chews-homemade-gin-gins**

National Library of Medicine / National Center for Biotechnology Information, Parojic, D., Stupar, D., Mirica, M., *Theriac: Medicine and Antidote*, **https://pubmed.ncbi.nlm.nih.gov/15125416**

National Library of Medicine / National Center for Biotechnology Information, Zargaran, A., Zarshenas, M., Mehdizadeh, A., and Mohagheghzadeh, A., *Oxymel in Medieval Persia*, **https://pubmed.ncbi.nlm.nih.gov/22530314**

Royal Botanic Gardens Kew, *Cacao Tree*, **https://kew.org/plants/cacao-tree**

Smithsonian Magazine, Sethi, S., *The Bittersweet Story of Vanilla*, **https://smithsonianmag.com/science-nature/bittersweet-story-vanilla-180962757**

Unruly Gardening, *How to Forage & Use Pine Resin*, **https://unrulygardening.com/forage-use-pine-resin**

Wellcome Collection, Jenner, E., *For Makeing of Waters and Syrups and Other Physical Remedies (1706)*, **https://wellcomecollection.org/works/ptkdwrp8**

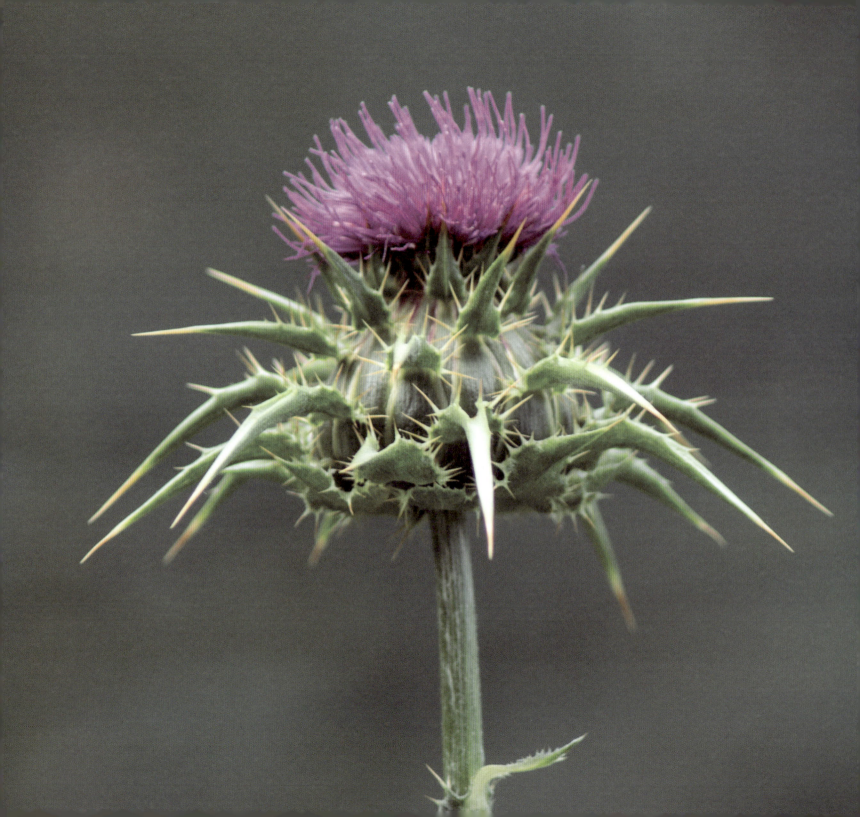

ACKNOWLEDGEMENTS & THANKS

WITH GRATITUDE

The beautiful imagery that accompanies the text has been diligently compiled by JACQUI PESTELL MBE, director of botanical illustration at the Garden, and KATE SOLTAN, our dedicated freelance photographer. They contributed tirelessly towards the completion of this book, and I wish to express my deepest gratitude and appreciation to them both.

I would also like to thank SARAH ROBERTS, SHARON TINGEY, JACK BAKER, LYNSEY WILSON & PETER CLARKE for their wonderful illustrations and photographs that appear in the book, and the PUBLICATIONS TEAM (PAULA BUSHELL, ANDREW LINDSAY, FRANKIE MATHIESON, CAROLINE MUIR, SARAH WORRALL & ALICE YOUNG) for their dedication and guidance.

Thanks also go to the following people, who have all contributed to the wonderful herbology programme we currently enjoy at the Royal Botanic Garden Edinburgh:

LEIGH MORRIS, former Royal Botanic Garden Edinburgh director of learning & horticulture, upon whose request the first herbology classes took place in the Garden – after hours.

SUZANNE HERMISTON, Royal Botanic Garden Edinburgh head of schools and online learning, for all her support of the herbology programme's development and for affording a book-writing sabbatical when it was most needed – twice.

DR GREG KENICER, Royal Botanic Garden Edinburgh head of graduate education and professional learning, our most erudite and much-published friend of herbology throughout the years.

MARTYN DICKSON, Royal Botanic Garden Edinburgh senior arboriculturist, one of herbology's most jovial followers since the very beginning, who has been the bearer of such a generous abundance of botanical ingredients from his travels to distant lands that he is now renown (to us) as the purveyor of some of the finest *Materia medica* we have ever had the pleasure to work with.

PHIL LUSBY, former Royal Botanic Garden Edinburgh director of garden history, botanist extraordinaire and connoisseur of fine roses, who has accompanied herbology groups on countless botanising expeditions out to East Lothian and most recently explained the more unfamiliar practices found within Evelyn's *Kalendarium*.

ANNA CANNING, Royal Botanic Garden Edinburgh herbology teaching assistant and most indispensable colleague.

DR MOONSIK CHANG, CEO at The Secrets of Caledonia, for his enduring and generous support of the Royal Botanic Garden Edinburgh's herbology programme.

DR MAUREEN MANSELL, anthropologist and herbologist, whose many untold treasures (often forwarded from Santa Fe) have uniquely enriched and informed the herbology programme.

PROFESSOR GORDON MANSELL, artist and adventurer, for his original 'Heath Robinson Affair' of a herbal percolator.

TOMAS ENOS, president of Milagro Herbs, Inc. in Santa Fe, for his generous sharing of Midwestern American herbal knowledge and dispatches of desert and sea formulations and percolation techniques. (The art of herbal percolation is taught as part of our Diploma in Herbology.)

IAIN MILNE, former head of heritage, Royal College of Physicians Edinburgh, for such colourful herbal anecdotes in the RCPE Sibbald Library over the years and for releasing one of only three precious copies of the first edition of the *Edinburgh Pharmacopoeia* (1699) for translation.

ROBERT MILL, Royal Botanic Garden Edinburgh research associate, for his enthusiastic translation of the first edition of the *Edinburgh Pharmacopoeia*, accomplished with such an extraordinary turn of speed and alacrity that we were beyond impressed, and whose scholarly example is something to which I can only aspire to!

ESTELA DUKAN, Royal College of Physicians Edinburgh Sibbald library staff, for all her help eliciting further details about the *Edinburgh Pharmacopoeia*.

GRAHAM HARDY, Royal Botanic Garden Edinburgh senior librarian, for facilitating access to archival records and publications, including Evelyn's *Kalendarium Hortense*, over an extended period.

KATE EDEN, SUZANNE CUBEY & LESLEY SCOTT, Royal Botanic Garden Edinburgh herbarium staff, for arranging herbology group viewings of the herbaria pressings of selected theriaca ingredients, and so much more.

FIONA INCHES, Royal Botanic Garden Edinburgh senior horticulturalist, for facilitating access to the glasshouses during biomes.

GUNNAR HARPER-OVSTEBO, Royal Botanic Garden Edinburgh arid lands glasshouse curator, for the best 'behind the scenes' glasshouse tours and Marley stories.

PAUL NESBITT, former Inverleith House curator of exhibitions, for first suggesting I meet with Leigh Morris.

The following herbology graduates and recipe contributors: SENGA BATE, my irreplaceable 'wing woman'; SUSAN RENNIE, for the most delicious lozenge recipe; CATHERINE SANDERSON, for her equally delicious croupy cough mixture; NICOLA TODD-MACNAUGHTON, for her beautiful distilled rose water cream; JACINTA NEGRI, diligent bonfire ginger toffee-maker; HEATHER POWER & CAISEY HOLLYWOOD, keen coltsfoot lozenge-makers; and to all our wonderful herbology VOLUNTEERS, VISITING LECTURERS, COLLEAGUES & COLLABORATORS, who have contributed so much.

And to all our kind friends of herbology, past and present, who have not been mentioned here but who dance with nature's spirits, thank you!

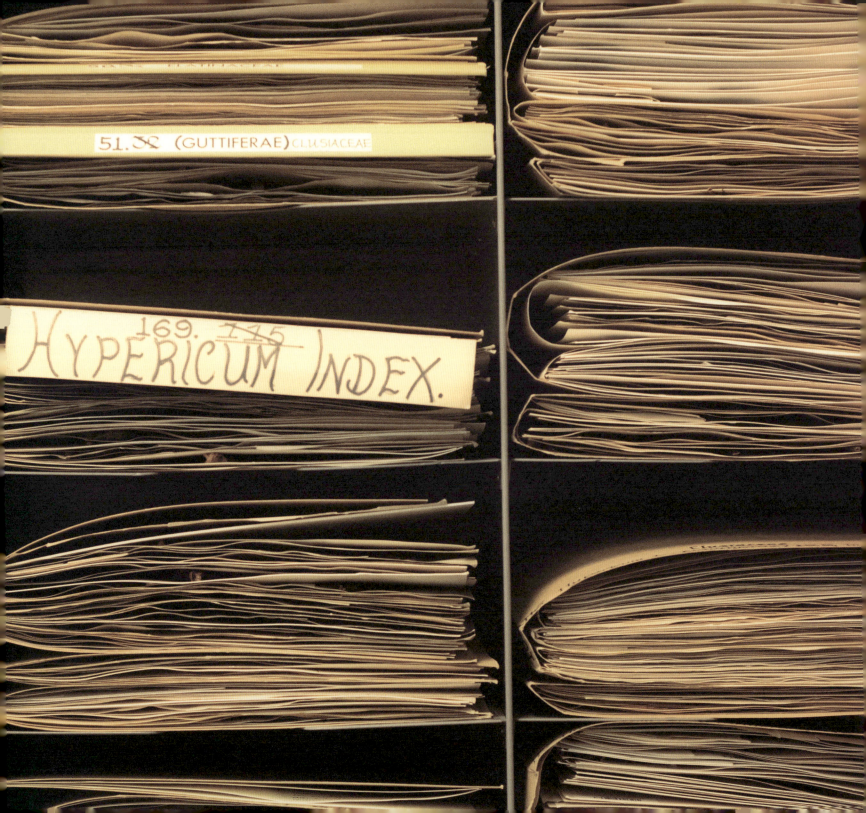

51.382 (GUTTIFERAE) CLUSIACEAE

169. 115
HYPERICUM INDEX.

INDEX

B

babies, and herbs 21

Bach, Edward, Dr 107

bain-marie 22

Balfour, Andrew 4

balm of Gilead buds (*Populus* x *gileadensis*) 176

balsams 218, 219

  see also benzoin

barley, pearl barley 62

Bartram, John 207

Bartram, Thomas, *Encyclopedia of Herbal Medicine* (1995, 1998) 35, 174

basil 27

bath powders *see* willow milk bath powders

bats 105

  pipistrelle bats 12

beans 136, 143

bee gum balm 231

bees 27, 86, 143

  honeybees 86, 141, 167

beeswax

  in benzoin vapour rub 227

  in blue chamomile balm 59

  in comfrey root balm 190

  in frozen winter bloom cream 208

  in green herb ointment 57

  in green herb-infused oil 54

  in ointments 56, 83

  in pine resin salve 229, 231

  in plasters 72

  in rose water cream 97

in yarrow-based balm ointment 37

beets 27

  beetroot powder 234

Bellis perennis (daisies) 35, 87, 108, 128

Beltane 25, 80, 122

Beltane flower cordial 31, 80

  recipe 81

benzoin

  benefits of 219

  benzoic acid 218

  recipes

    alcoholic extract of benzoin 222

    benzoin vapour rub 227

    benzoin-infused oil 221

    oil of benzoin embrocation 224

    oil of benzoin liniment 225

Berberis 146

bergamot oil 124, 125

Betula pendula (birch) 43

bicarbonate of soda 133, 134, 135

bilberry 155, 159

biodiversity crisis 5

biodynamic horticulture 12

birch (*Betula pendula*) 43

bistort 33, 62

black lace elder (*Sambucus nigra*) 113

black salsify 27

black strap molasses 61

black truffle fungi (*Tuber melanosporum*) 233

blackberries 141, 155, 159, 168, 181

blackcurrants (*Ribes nigrum*) 42, 86, 113, 141, 160, 168, 181

blackthorns 25, 33

blaeberries 181

blenders 22

blood clotting/thinning 199

blood pressure (high) 39

bloodwort *see* St John's wort (*Hypericum perforatum*)

bloom cream *see* frozen winter bloom cream

blueberries 136

bogbean 77

bonfire ginger root toffee 197

  recipe 212–13

borage (*Borago officinalis*) 27, 113

botanic gardens

  first ones 14

  see also Royal Botanic Garden Edinburgh (RBGE)

botanical medicine *see* medicinal botany

brandy 146, 200

breastfeeding, and herbs 21

British Pimm's 113

bruisewort *see* daisies (*Bellis perennis*)

bryony root (*Bryonia dioica*) 136

buckthorn oil 77

Bufo exsiccatus (powdered toad) 9

bugloss 27

bulbs

  autumn bulbs 87, 143

  flowering bulbs 13

butters

  cocoa butter 97

  shea butter 97

  stockist 23

C

F

G

H

I

J

K

L

W

Y

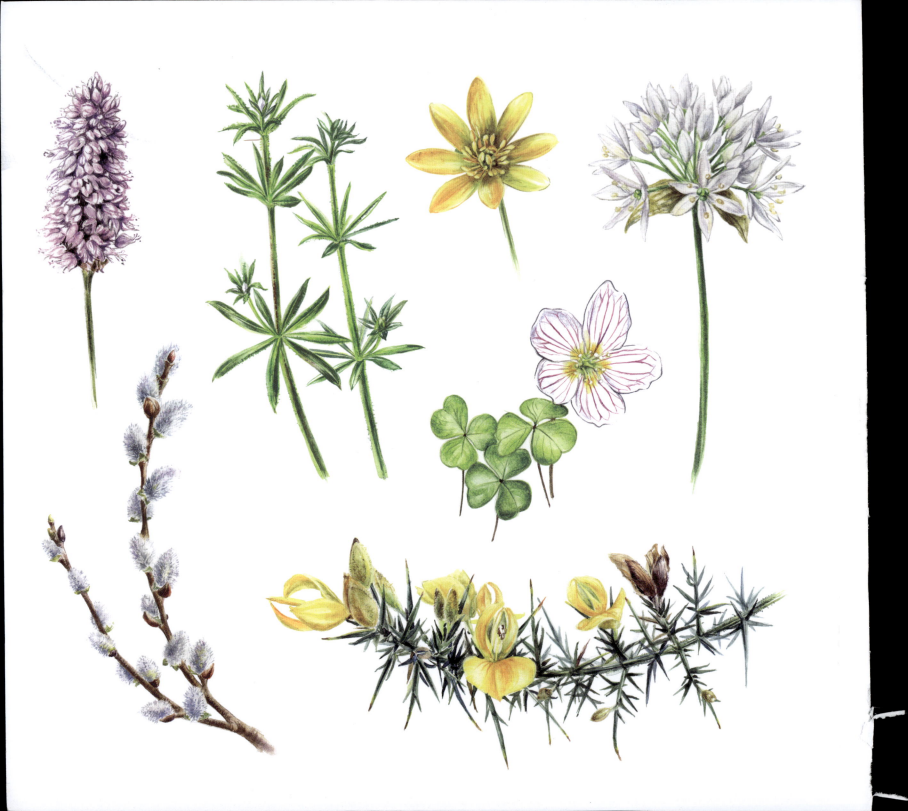